Virtual Clinical Excursions—Obstetrics

for

Lowdermilk and Perry:
Maternity and Women's Health Care,
9th Edition

Virtual Clinical Excursions—Obstetrics

for

Lowdermilk and Perry:
Maternity and Women's Health Care,
9th Edition

prepared by

Kitty Cashion, RN, BC, MSN
Clinical Nurse Specialist
University of Tennessee, Memphis, Health Science Center
Department of Obstetrics and Gynecology
Division of Maternal-Fetal Medicine
Memphis, Tennessee

Kelly Ann Crum, RN, MSN
Instructional Specialist
Lead Faculty
Curriculum Development/Maternal Child Nursing Specialty
Health Sciences and Nursing Department
University of Phoenix, Online
Phoenix, Arizona

software developed by

Wolfsong Informatics, LLC
Tucson, Arizona

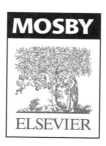

MOSBY

ELSEVIER

11830 Westline Industrial Dr.
St. Louis, Missouri 63146

VIRTUAL CLINICAL EXCURSIONS—OBSTETRICS FOR
LOWDERMILK AND PERRY: MATERNITY AND WOMEN'S HEALTH CARE
NINTH EDITION
Copyright © 2007 by Mosby, Inc., an affiliate of Elsevier Inc.

Notice

Knowledge and best practice in this field are constantly changing. As new research and experience broaden our knowledge, changes in practice, treatment and drug therapy may become necessary or appropriate. Readers are advised to check the most current information provided (i) on procedures featured or (ii) by the manufacturer of each product to be administered, to verify the recommended dose or formula, the method and duration of administration, and contraindications. It is the responsibility of the practitioner, relying on their own experience and knowledge of the patient, to make diagnoses, to determine dosages and the best treatment for each individual patient, and to take all appropriate safety precautions. To the fullest extent of the law, neither the Publisher nor the Authors assumes any liability for any injury and/or damage to persons or property arising out or related to any use of the material contained in this book.

ISBN-13: 978-0-323-05016-6
ISBN-10: 0-323-05016-6

Executive Editor: *Tom Wilhelm*
Managing Editor: *Jeff Downing*
Associate Developmental Editor: *Tiffany Trautwein*
Book Production Manager: *Gayle May*
Project Manager: *Tracey Schriefer*

Printed in the United States of America

Last digit is the print number: 9   8   7   6   5   4

Workbook
prepared by

Kitty Cashion, RN, BC, MSN
Clinical Nurse Specialist
University of Tennessee, Memphis, Health Science Center
Department of Obstetrics and Gynecology
Division of Maternal-Fetal Medicine
Memphis, Tennessee

Kelly Ann Crum, RN, MSN
Instructional Specialist
Lead Faculty
Curriculum Development/Maternal Child Nursing Specialty
Health Sciences and Nursing Department
University of Phoenix, Online
Phoenix, Arizona

Textbook

Deitra Leonard Lowdermilk, RNC, PhD, FAAN
Clinical Professor, School of Nursing
Nursing Education and Curriculum Consultant
University of North Carolina at Chapel Hill
Chapel Hill, North Carolina

Shannon E. Perry, RN, CNS, PhD, FAAN
Professor Emerita, School of Nursing
San Francisco State University
San Francisco, California

Contents

Table of Contents
Lowdermilk and Perry:
Maternity and Women's Health Care, 9th Edition

Getting Started

GETTING SET UP

■ **MINIMUM SYSTEM REQUIREMENTS**

WINDOWS®

Windows Vista™, XP, 2000 (Recommend Windows XP/2000)
Pentium® III processor (or equivalent) @ 600 MHz (Recommend 800 MHz or better)
256 MB of RAM (Recommend 1 GB or more for Windows Vista)
800 x 600 screen size (Recommend 1024 x 768)
Thousands of colors
12x CD-ROM drive
Soundblaster 16 soundcard compatibility
Stereo speakers or headphones

Note: Windows Vista and XP require administrator privileges for installation.

MACINTOSH®

MAC OS X (10.2 or higher)
Apple Power PC G3 @ 500 MHz or better
128 MB of RAM (Recommend 256 MB or more)
800 x 600 screen size (Recommend 1024 x 768)
Thousands of colors
12x CD-ROM drive
Stereo speakers or headphones

■ INSTALLATION INSTRUCTIONS

WINDOWS

1. Insert the *Virtual Clinical Excursions—Obstetrics* CD-ROM.
2. The setup screen should appear automatically if the current product is not already installed. Windows Vista users may be asked to authorize additional security prompts.
3. Follow the onscreen instructions during the setup process.

If the setup screen does *not* appear automatically (and *Virtual Clinical Excursions— Obstetrics* has not been installed already):
a. Click the **My Computer** icon on your desktop or on your Start menu.
b. Double-click on your CD-ROM drive.
c. If installation does not start at this point:
   (1) Click the **Start** icon on the taskbar and select the **Run** option.
   (2) Type d:\setup.exe (where "d:\" is your CD-ROM drive) and press **OK**.
   (3) Follow the onscreen instructions for installation.

MACINTOSH

1. Insert the *Virtual Clinical Excursions—Obstetrics* CD in the CD-ROM drive. The disk icon will appear on your desktop.

2. Double-click on the disk icon.

3. Double-click on the OBSTETRICS_MAC run file.

Note: Virtual Clinical Excursions—Obstetrics for Macintosh does not have an installation setup and can only be run directly from the CD.

■ HOW TO USE VIRTUAL CLINICAL EXCURSIONS—OBSTETRICS

WINDOWS

1. Double-click on the *Virtual Clinical Excursions—Obstetrics* icon located on your desktop.
2. Or navigate to the program via the Windows Start menu.

Note: If your computer uses Windows Vista, right-click on the desktop shortcut and choose **Properties**. In the Compatability Mode, check the box for "Run as Administrator." Below is a screen capture to show what this looks like.

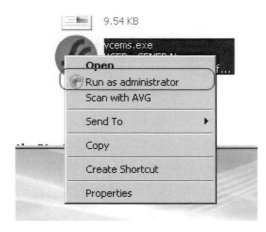

■ **MACINTOSH**

1. Insert the *Virtual Clinical Excursions—Obstetrics* CD in the CD-ROM drive. The disk icon will appear on your desktop.
2. Double-click on the disk icon.
3. Double-click on the OBSTETRICS_MAC run file.

SCREEN SETTINGS

For best results, your computer monitor resolution should be set at a minimum of 800 x 600. The number of colors displayed should be set to "thousands or higher" (High Color or 16 bit) or "millions of colors" (True Color or 24 bit).

Windows

1. From the **Start** menu, select **Control Panel** (on some systems, you will first go to **Settings**, then to **Control Panel**).
2. Double-click on the **Display** icon.
3. Click on the **Settings** tab.
4. Under **Screen resolution** use the slider bar to select **800 by 600 pixels**.
5. Access the **Colors** drop-down menu by clicking on the down arrow.
6. Select **High Color (16 bit)** or **True Color (24 bit)**.
7. Click on **OK**.
8. You may be asked to verify the setting changes. Click **Yes**.
9. You may be asked to restart your computer to accept the changes. Click **Yes**.

Macintosh

1. Select the **Monitors** control panel.
2. Select **800 x 600** (or similar) from the **Resolution** area.
3. Select **Thousands** or **Millions** from the **Color Depth** area.

■ WEB BROWSERS

Supported web browsers include Microsoft Internet Explorer (IE) version 6.0 or higher and Mozilla Firefox version 2.0 or higher. The supported browser for Macs running OS X is Mozilla Firefox.

If you use America Online® (AOL) for web access, you will need AOL version 4.0 or higher and one of the browsers listed above. Do not use earlier versions of AOL with earlier versions of IE, because you will have difficulty accessing many features.

For best results with AOL:
- Connect to the Internet using AOL version 4.0 or higher.
- Open a private chat within AOL (this allows the AOL client to remain open, without asking whether you wish to disconnect while minimized).
- Minimize AOL.
- Launch a recommended browser.

■ TECHNICAL SUPPORT

Technical support for this product is available between 7:30 a.m. and 7 p.m. (CST), Monday through Friday. Before calling, be sure that your computer meets the minimum system requirements to run this software. Inside the United States and Canada, call 1-800-692-9010. Outside North America, call 314-872-8370. You may also fax your questions to 314-523-4932 or contact Technical Support through e-mail: technical.support@elsevier.com.

Trademarks: Windows, Macintosh, Pentium, and America Online are registered trademarks.

Copyright © 2007 by Mosby, Inc., an affiliate of Elsevier Inc.

ACCESSING *Virtual Clinical Excursions—Obstetrics* FROM EVOLVE

The product you have purchased is part of the Evolve family of online courses and learning resources. Please read the following information thoroughly to get started.

To access your instructor's course on Evolve:

Your instructor will provide you with the username and password needed to access this specific course on the Evolve Learning System. Once you have received this information, please follow these instructions:

1. Go to the Evolve student page (http://evolve.elsevier.com/student).

2. Enter your username and password in the **Login to My Evolve** area and click the **Login** button.

3. You will be taken to your personalized **My Evolve** page, where the course will be listed in the **My Courses** module.

TECHNICAL REQUIREMENTS

To use an Evolve course, you will need access to a computer that is connected to the Internet and equipped with web browser software that supports frames. For optimal performance, it is recommended that you have speakers and use a high-speed Internet connection. However, slower dial-up modems (56 K minimum) are acceptable.

Whichever browser you use, the browser preferences must be set to enable cookies and JavaScript and the cache must be set to reload every time.

Enable Cookies

Browser	Steps
Internet Explorer (IE) 6.0 or higher	1. Select **Tools → Internet Options**. 2. Select **Privacy** tab. 3. Use the slider (slide down) to **Accept All Cookies**. 4. Click **OK**. -OR- 3. Click the **Advanced** button. 4. Click the check box next to **Override Automatic Cookie Handling**. 5. Click the **Accept** radio buttons under **First-party Cookies** and **Third-party Cookies**. 6. Click **OK**.
Mozilla Firefox 2.0 or higher	1. Select **Tools → Options**. 2. Select the **Privacy** icon. 3. Click to expand Cookies. 4. Select **Allow sites to set cookies**. 5. Click **OK**.

Set Cache to Always Reload a Page

Browser	Steps
Internet Explorer (IE) 6.0 or higher	1. Select **Tools → Internet Options**. 2. Select **General** tab. 3. Go to the **Temporary Internet Files** and click the **Settings** button. 4. Select the radio button for **Every visit to the page** and click **OK** when complete.
Mozilla Firefox 2.0 or higher	1. Select **Tools → Options**. 2. Select the **Privacy** icon. 3. Click to expand Cache. 4. Set the value to "**0**" in the **Use up to: __ MB of disk space for the cache** field. 5. Click **OK**.

Plug-Ins

 Adobe Acrobat Reader—With the free Acrobat Reader software, you can view and print Adobe PDF files. Many Evolve products offer student and instructor manuals, checklists, and more in this format!

Download at: http://www.adobe.com

 Apple QuickTime—Install this to hear word pronunciations, heart and lung sounds, and many other helpful audio clips within Evolve Online Courses!

Download at: http://www.apple.com

 Adobe Flash Player—This player will enhance your viewing of many Evolve web pages, as well as educational short-form to long-form animation within the Evolve Learning System!

Download at: http://www.adobe.com

 Adobe Shockwave Player—Shockwave is best for viewing the many interactive learning activities within Evolve Online Courses!

Download at: http://www.adobe.com

 Microsoft Word Viewer—With this viewer, Microsoft Word users can share documents with those who don't have Word, and users without Word can open and view Word documents. Many Evolve products have testbank, student and instructor manuals, and other documents available for downloading and viewing on your own computer!

Download at: http://www.microsoft.com

 Microsoft PowerPoint Viewer—With this viewer, you can access PowerPoint 97, 2000, and 2002 presentations even if you don't have PowerPoint. Many Evolve products have slides available for downloading and viewing on your own computer!

Download at: http://www.microsoft.com

SUPPORT INFORMATION

Live phone support is available to customers in the United States and Canada at **800-401-9962** from 7:30 a.m. to 7 p.m. (CST), Monday through Friday. Support is also available through email at evolve-support@elsevier.com.

Online 24/7 support can be accessed on the Evolve website (http://evolve.elsevier.com). Resources include:

- Guided tours
- Tutorials
- Frequently asked questions (FAQs)
- Online copies of course user guides
- And much more!

A QUICK TOUR

Welcome to *Virtual Clinical Excursions—Obstetrics*, a virtual hospital setting in which you can work with multiple complex patient simulations and also learn to access and evaluate the information resources that are essential for high-quality patient care. The virtual hospital, Pacific View Regional Hospital, has realistic architecture and access to patient rooms, a Nurses' Station, and a Medication Room.

■ BEFORE YOU START

Make sure you have your textbook nearby when you use the *Virtual Clinical Excursions— Obstetrics* CD. You will want to consult topic areas in your textbook frequently while working with the CD and using this workbook.

■ HOW TO SIGN IN

- Enter your name on the Student Nurse identification badge.
- Now choose one of the four periods of care in which to work. In Periods of Care 1 through 3, you can actively engage in patient assessment, entry of data in the electronic patient record (EPR), and medication administration. Period of Care 4 presents the day in review. Click on the appropriate period of care. (For this quick tour, choose **Period of Care 1: 0730-0815**.)
- This takes you to the Patient List screen (see example on page 11). Note that the virtual time is provided in the box at the lower left corner of the screen (0730, since we chose Period of Care 1).

Note: If you choose to work during Period of Care 4: 1900-2000, the Patient List screen is skipped since you are not able to visit patients or administer medications during the shift. Instead, you are taken directly to the Nurses' Station, where the records of all the patients on the floor are available for your review.

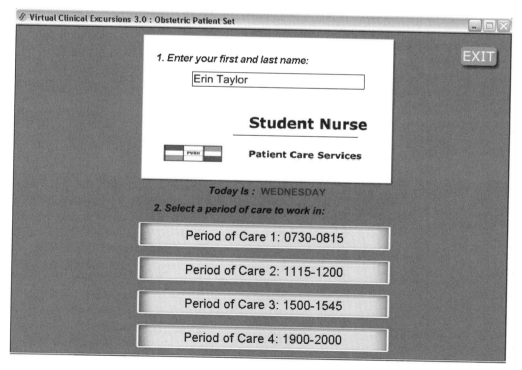

■ PATIENT LIST

Obstetrics Unit

Dorothy Grant (Room 201)
30-week intrauterine pregnancy—A 25-year-old Caucasian multipara admitted with abdominal trauma following a domestic violence incident. Her complications include preterm labor and extensive social issues such as acquiring safe housing for her family upon discharge.

Stacey Crider (Room 202)
27-week intrauterine pregnancy—A 21-year-old Native American primigravida admitted for intravenous tocolysis, bacterial vaginosis, and poorly controlled insulin-dependent gestational diabetes. Strained family relationships and social isolation complicate this patient's ability to comply with strict dietary requirements and prenatal care.

Kelly Brady (Room 203)
26-week intrauterine pregnancy—A 35-year-old Caucasian primigravida urgently admitted for progressive symptoms of preeclampsia. A history of inadequate coping with major life stressors leave her at risk for a recurrence of depression as she faces a diagnosis of HELLP syndrome and the delivery of a severely premature infant.

Maggie Gardner (Room 204)
22-week intrauterine pregnancy—A 41-year-old African-American multigravida admitted for a high-risk pregnancy evaluation and rule out diagnosis of systemic lupus erythematosus. Coping with chronic pain, fatigue, and a history of multiple miscarriages contribute to an anxiety disorder and the need for social service intervention.

Gabriela Valenzuela (Room 205)
34-week intrauterine pregnancy—A 21-year-old Hispanic primigravida with a history of mitral valve prolapse admitted for uterine cramping and vaginal bleeding suggestive of placental abruption following an unrestrained motor vehicle accident. Her needs include staff support for an unprepared-for labor and possible preterm birth.

Laura Wilson (Room 206)
37-week intrauterine pregnancy—An 18-year-old Caucasian primigravida urgently admitted after being found unconscious at home. Her complications include HIV-positive status and chronic polysubstance abuse. Unrealistic expectations of parenthood and living with a chronic illness combined with strained family relations prompt comprehensive social and psychiatric evaluations initiated on the day of simulation.

■ HOW TO SELECT A PATIENT

- You can choose one or more patients to work with from the Patient List by checking the box to the left of the patient name(s). For this quick tour, select Dorothy Grant. (In order to receive a scorecard for a patient, the patient must be selected before proceeding to the Nurses' Station.)
- Click on **Get Report** to the right of the medical records number (MRN) to view a summary of the patient's care during the 12-hour period before your arrival on the unit.
- After reviewing the report, click on **Go to Nurses' Station** in the right lower corner to begin your care. (*Note:* If you have been assigned to care for multiple patients, you can click on **Return to Patient List** to select and review the report for each additional patient before going to the Nurses' Station.)

Note: Even though the Patient List is initially skipped when you sign in to work for Period of Care 4, you can still access this screen if you wish to review the shift report for any of the patients. To do so, simply click on **Patient List** near the top left corner of the Nurses' Station (or click on the clipboard to the left of the Kardex). Then click on **Get Report** for the patient(s) whose care you are reviewing. This may be done during any period of care.

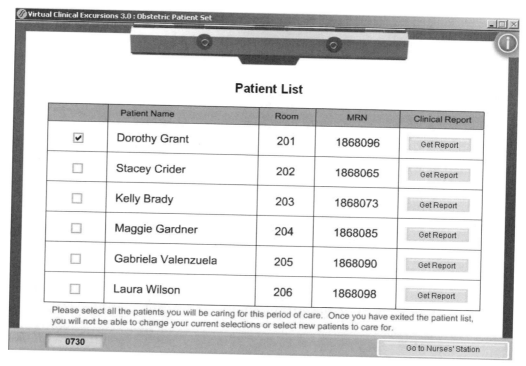

■ HOW TO FIND A PATIENT'S RECORDS

NURSES' STATION

Within the Nurses' Station, you will see:

1. A clipboard that contains the patient list for that floor.
2. A chart rack with patient charts labeled by room number, a notebook labeled Kardex, and a notebook labeled MAR (Medication Administration Record).
3. A desktop computer with access to the Electronic Patient Record (EPR).
4. A tool bar across the top of the screen that can also be used to access the Patient List, EPR, Chart, MAR, and Kardex. This tool bar is also accessible from each patient's room.
5. A Drug Guide containing information about the medications you are able to administer to your patients.
6. A tool bar across the bottom of the screen that can be used to access the Floor Map, patient rooms, Medication Room, and Drug Guide.

As you run your cursor over an item, it will be highlighted. To select, simply double-click on the item. As you use these resources, you will always be able to return to the Nurses' Station by clicking on the **Return to Nurses' Station** bar located in the right lower corner of your screen.

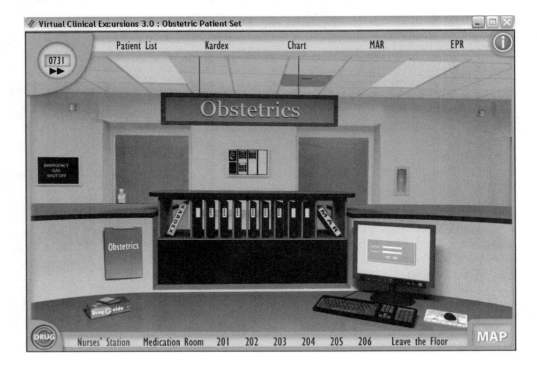

MEDICATION ADMINISTRATION RECORD (MAR)

The MAR icon located on the tool bar at the top of your screen accesses current 24-hour medications for each patient. Click on the icon and the MAR will open. (*Note:* You can also access the MAR by clicking on the MAR notebook on the far right side of the book rack in the center of the screen.) Within the MAR, tabs on the right side of the screen allow you to select patients by room number. Be careful to make sure you select the correct tab number for *your* patient rather than simply reading the first record that appears after the MAR opens. Each MAR sheet lists the following:

- Medications
- Route and dosage of each medication
- Times of administration of each medication

Note: The MAR changes each day. Expired MARs are stored in the patients' charts.

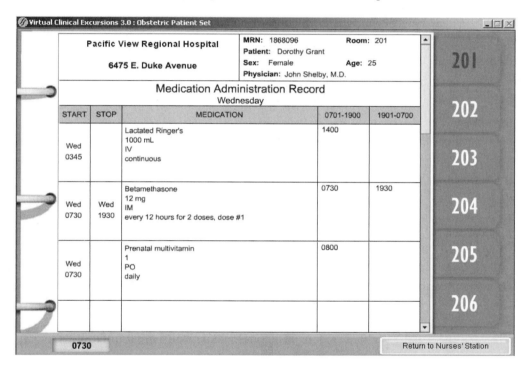

CHARTS

To access patient charts, either click on the **Chart** icon at the top of your screen or anywhere within the chart rack in the center of the Nurses' Station screen. When the close-up view appears, the individual charts are labeled by room number. To open a chart, click on the room number of the patient whose chart you wish to review. The patient's name and allergies will appear on the left side of the screen, along with a list of tabs on the right side of the screen, allowing you to view the following data:

- Allergies
- Physician's Orders
- Physician's Notes
- Nurse's Notes
- Laboratory Reports
- Diagnostic Reports
- Surgical Reports
- Consultations

- Patient Education
- History and Physical
- Nursing Admission
- Expired MARs
- Consents
- Mental Health
- Admissions
- Emergency Department

Information appears in real time. The entries are in reverse chronologic order, so use the down arrow at the right side of each chart page to scroll down to view previous entries. Flip from tab to tab to view multiple data fields or click on **Return to Nurses' Station** in the lower right corner of the screen to exit the chart.

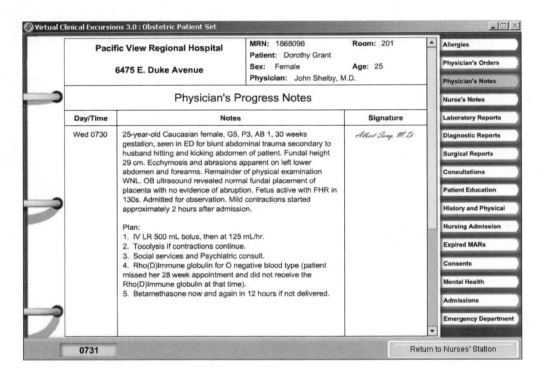

ELECTRONIC PATIENT RECORD (EPR)

The EPR can be accessed from the computer in the Nurses' Station or from the EPR icon located in the tool bar at the top of your screen. To access a patient's EPR:

- Click on either the computer screen or the **EPR** icon.
- Your username and password are automatically filled in.
- Click on **Login** to enter the EPR.
- *Note:* Like the MAR, the EPR is arranged numerically. Thus when you enter, you are initially shown the records of the patient in the lowest room number on the floor. To view the correct data for *your* patient, remember to select the correct room number, using the drop-down menu for the Patient field at the top left corner of the screen.

The EPR used in Pacific View Regional Hospital represents a composite of commercial versions being used in hospitals. You can access the EPR:

- to review existing data for a patient (by room number).
- to enter data you collect while working with a patient.

The EPR is updated daily, so no matter what day or part of a shift you are working, there will be a current EPR with the patient's data from the past days of the current hospital stay. This type of simulated EPR allows you to examine how data for different attributes have changed over time, as well as to examine data for all of a patient's attributes at a particular time. The EPR is fully functional (as it is in a real-life hospital). You can enter such data as blood pressure, breath sounds, and certain treatments. The EPR will not, however, allow you to enter data for a previous time period. Use the arrows at the bottom of the screen to move forward and backward in time.

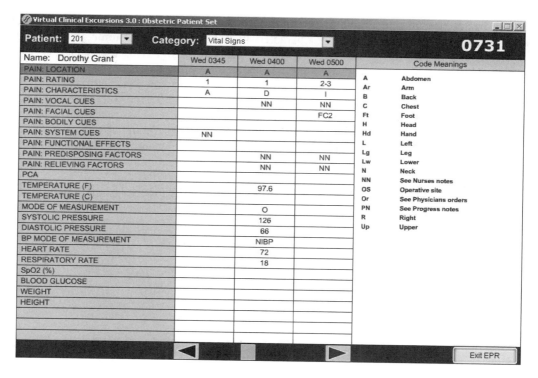

At the top of the EPR screen, you can choose patients by their room numbers. In addition, you have access to 17 different categories of patient data. To change patients or data categories, click the down arrow to the right of the room number or category.

The categories of patient data in the EPR as as follows:

- Vital Signs
- Respiratory
- Cardiovascular
- Neurologic
- Gastrointestinal
- Excretory
- Musculoskeletal
- Integumentary
- Reproductive
- Psychosocial
- Wounds and Drains
- Activity
- Hygiene and Comfort
- Safety
- Nutrition
- IV
- Intake and Output

Remember, each hospital selects its own codes. The codes used in the EPR at Pacific View Regional Hospital may be different from ones you have seen in your clinical rotations. Take some time to acquaint yourself with the codes. Within the Vital Signs category, click on any item in the left column (e.g., Pain: Characteristics). In the far-right column, you will see a list of code meanings for the possible findings and/or descriptors for that assessment area.

You will use the codes to record the data you collect as you work with patients. Click on the box in the last time column to the right of any item and wait for the code meanings applicable to that entry to appear. Select the appropriate code to describe your assessment findings and type it in the box. (*Note:* If no cursor appears within the box, click on the box again until the blue shading disappears and the blinking cursor appears.) Once the data are typed in this box, they are entered into the patient's record for this period of care only.

To leave the EPR, click on **Exit EPR** in the bottom right corner of the screen.

■ VISITING A PATIENT

From the Nurses' Station, click on the room number of the patient you wish to visit (in the tool bar at the bottom of your screen). Once you are inside the room, you will see a still photo of your patient in the top left corner. To verify that this is the correct patient, click on the **Check Armband** icon to the right of the photo. The patient's identification data will appear. If you click on **Check Allergies** (the next icon to the right), a list of the patient's allergies (if any) will replace the photo.

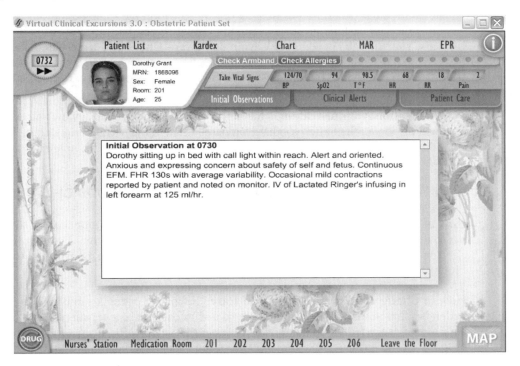

Also located in the patient's room are multiple icons you can use to assess the patient or the patient's medications. A virtual clock is provided in the upper left corner of the room to monitor your progress in real time. (*Note:* The fast-forward icon within the virtual clock will advance the time by 2-minute intervals when clicked.)

- The tool bar across the top of the screen allows you to check the **Patient List**, access the **EPR** to check or enter data, and view the patient's **Chart**, **MAR**, or **Kardex**.

- The **Take Vital Signs** icon allows you to measure the patient's up-to-the-minute blood pressure, oxygen saturation, temperature, heart rate, respiratory rate, and pain level.

- Each time you enter a patient's room, you are given an Initial Observation report to review (in the text box under the patient's photo). These notes are provided to give you a "look" at the patient as if you had just stepped into the room. You can also click on the **Initial Observations** icon to return to this box from other views within the patient's room. To the right of this icon is **Clinical Alerts**, a resource that allows you to make decisions about priority medication interventions based on emerging data collected in real time. Check this screen throughout your period of care to avoid missing critical information related to recently ordered or STAT medications.

- Clicking on **Patient Care** opens up three specific learning environments within the patient room: **Physical Assessment**, **Nurse-Client Interactions**, and **Medication Administration**.

- To perform a **Physical Assessment**, choose a body area (such as **Head & Neck**) from the column of yellow buttons. This activates a list of system subcategories for that body area (e.g., see **Sensory**, **Neurologic**, etc. in the green boxes). After you select the system you wish to evaluate, a brief description of the assessment findings will appear in a box to the right. A still photo provides a "snapshot" of how an assessment of this area might be done or what the finding might look like. For every body area, you can also click on **Equipment** on the right side of the screen.

- To the right of the Physical Assessment icon is **Nurse-Client Interactions**. Clicking on this icon will reveal the times and titles of any videos available for viewing. (*Note:* If the video you wish to see is not listed, this means you have not yet reached the correct virtual time to view that video. Check the virtual clock; you may return to access the video once its designated time has occurred—as long as you do so within the same period of care. Or you can click on the fast-forward icon within the virtual clock to advance the time by 2-minute intervals. You will then need to click again on **Patient Care** and **Nurse-Client Interactions** to refresh the screen.) To view a listed video, click on the white arrow to the right of the video title. Use the control buttons below the video to start, stop, pause, rewind, or fast-forward the action or to mute the sound.

- **Medication Administration** is the pathway that allows you to review and administer medications to a patient after you have prepared them in the Medication Room. This process is addressed further in *How to Prepare Medications* (pages 19-20), in *Medications* (pages 26-30), and in *Reducing Medication Errors* (pages 37-41).

■ HOW TO QUIT, CHANGE PATIENTS, OR CHANGE PERIODS OF CARE

How to Quit: From most screens, you may click the **Leave the Floor** icon on the bottom tool bar to the right of the patient room numbers. (*Note:* From some screens, you will first need to click an **Exit** button or **Return to Nurses' Station** before clicking **Leave the Floor**.) When the Floor Menu appears, click **Exit** to leave the program.

How to Change Patients or Periods of Care: To change patients, simply click on the new patient's room number. (You cannot receive a scorecard for a new patient, however, unless you have already selected that patient on the Patient List screen.) To change to a new period of care or to restart the virtual clock, click on **Leave the Floor** and then on **Restart the Program**.

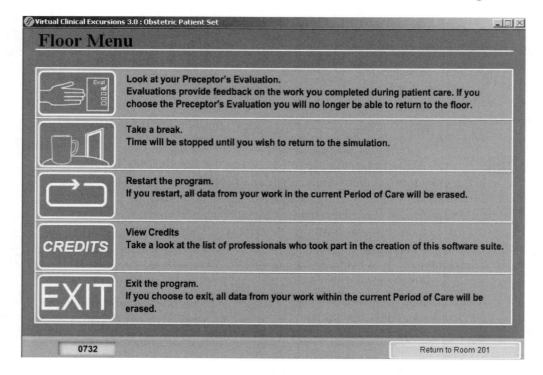

■ HOW TO PREPARE MEDICATIONS

From the Nurses' Station or the patient's room, you can access the Medication Room by clicking on the icon in the tool bar at the bottom of your screen to the left of the patient room numbers.

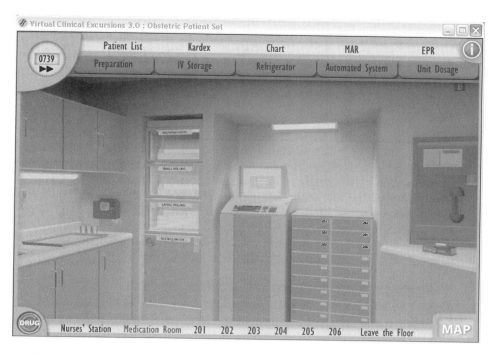

In the Medication Room you have access to the following (from left to right):

- A preparation area is located on the counter under the cabinets. To begin the medication preparation process, click on the tray on the counter or click on the **Preparation** icon at the top of the screen. The next screen leads you through a specific sequence (called the Preparation Wizard) to prepare medications one at a time for administration to a patient. However, no medication has been selected at this time. We will do this while working with a patient in *A Detailed Tour*. To exit this screen, click on **View Medication Room**.

- To the right of the cabinets (and above the refrigerator), IV storage bins are provided. Click on the bins themselves or on the **IV Storage** icon at the top of the screen. The bins are labeled **Microinfusion**, **Small Volume**, and **Large Volume**. Click on an individual bin to see a list of its contents. If you needed to prepare an IV medication at this time, you could click on the medication and its label would appear to the right under the patient's name. (*Note:* You can **Open** and **Close** any medication label by clicking the appropriate icon.) Next, you would click **Put Medication on Tray**. If you ever change your mind or decide that you have put the incorrect medication on the tray, you can reverse your actions by highlighting the medication on the tray and then clicking **Put Medication in Bin**. Click **Close Bin** in the right bottom corner to exit. **View Medication Room** brings you back to a full view of the entire room.

- A refrigerator is located under the IV storage bins to hold any medications that must be stored below room temperature. Click on the refrigerator door or on the **Refrigerator** icon at the top of the screen. Then click on the close-up view of the door to access the medications. When you are finished, click **Close Door** and then **View Medication Room**.

- To prepare controlled substances, click the **Automated System** icon at the top of the screen or click the computer monitor located to the right of the IV storage bins. A login screen will appear; your name and password are automatically filled in. Click **Login**. Select the patient for whom you wish to access medications; then select the correct medication drawer to open (they are stored alphabetically). Click **Open Drawer**, highlight the proper medication, and choose **Put Medication on Tray**. When you are finished, click **Close Drawer** and then **View Medication Room**.

- Next to the Automated System is a set of drawers identified by patient room number. To access these, click on the drawers or on the **Unit Dosage** icon at the top of the screen. This provides a close-up view of the drawers. To open a drawer, click on the room number of the patient you are working with. Next, click on the medication you would like to prepare for the patient, and a label will appear, listing the medication strength, units, and dosage per unit. To exit, click **Close Drawer**; then click **View Medication Room**.

At any time, you can learn about a medication you wish to prepare for a patient by clicking on the **Drug** icon in the bottom left corner of the medication room screen or by clicking the **Drug Guide** book on the counter to the right of the unit dosage drawers. The **Drug Guide** provides information about the medications commonly included in nursing drug handbooks. Nutritional supplements and maintenance intravenous fluid preparations are not included. Highlight a medication in the alphabetical list; relevant information about the drug will appear in the screen below. To exit, click **Return to Medication Room**.

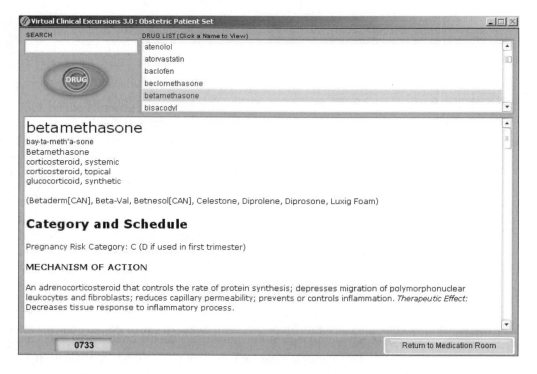

To access the MAR to review the medications ordered for a patient, click on the **MAR** icon located in the tool bar at the top of your screen and then click on the correct tab for your patient's room number. You may also click the **Review MAR** icon in the tool bar at the bottom of your screen from inside each medication storage area.

After you have chosen and prepared medications, go to the patient's room to administer them by clicking on the room number in the bottom tool bar. Inside the patient's room, click **Patient Care** and then **Medication Administration** and follow the proper administration sequence.

■ PRECEPTOR'S EVALUATIONS

When you have finished a session, click on **Leave the Floor** to go to the Floor Menu. At this point, you can click on the top icon (**Look at Your Preceptor's Evaluation**) to receive a score-card that provides feedback on the work you completed during patient care.

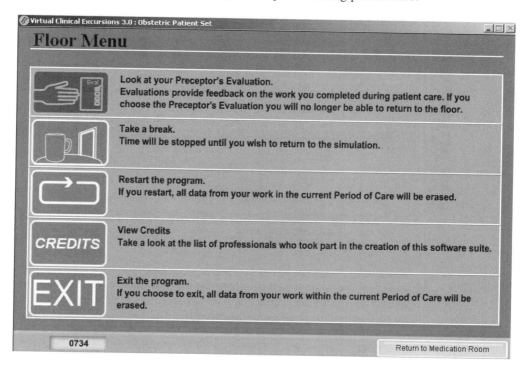

Evaluations are available for each patient you selected when you signed in for the current period of care. Click on the **Medication Scorecard** icon to see an example.

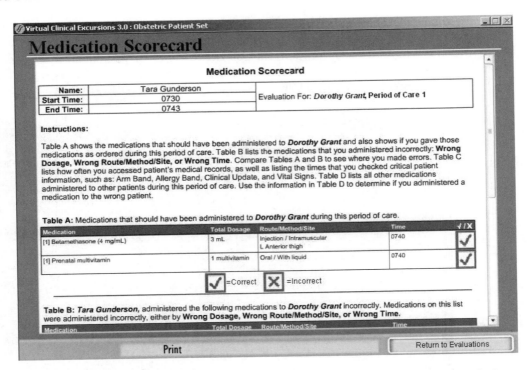

The scorecard compares the medications you administered to a patient during a period of care with what should have been administered. Table A lists the correct medications. Table B lists any medications that were administered incorrectly.

Remember, not every medication listed on the MAR should necessarily be given. For example, a patient might have an allergy to a drug that was ordered, or a medication might have been improperly transcribed to the MAR. Predetermined medication "errors" embedded within the program challenge you to exercise critical thinking skills and professional judgment when deciding to administer a medication, just as you would in a real hospital. Use all your available resources, such as the patient's chart and the MAR, to make your decision.

Table C lists the resources that were available to assist you in medication administration. It also documents whether and when you accessed these resources. For example, did you check the patient armband or perform a check of vital signs? If so, when?

You can click **Print** to get a copy of this report if needed. When you have finished reviewing the scorecard, click **Return to Evaluations** and then **Return to Menu**.

■ FLOOR MAP

To get a general sense of your location within the hospital, you can click on the **Map** icon found in the lower right corner of most of the screens in the *Virtual Clinical Excursions—Obstetrics* program. (*Note:* If you are following this quick tour step by step, you will need to **Restart the Program** from the Floor Menu, sign in again, and go to the Nurses' Station to access the map.) When you click the **Map** icon, a floor map appears, showing the layout of the floor you are currently on, as well as a directory of the patients and services on that floor. As you move your cursor over the directory list, the location of each room is highlighted on the map (and vice versa). The floor map can be accessed from the Nurses' Station, Medication Room, and each patient's room.

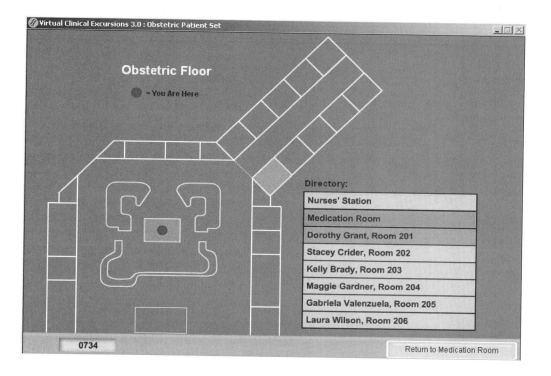

A DETAILED TOUR

If you wish to more thoroughly understand the capabilities of *Virtual Clinical Excursions—Obstetrics*, take a detailed tour by completing the following section. During this tour, we will work with a specific patient to introduce you to all the different components and learning opportunities available within the software.

■ WORKING WITH A PATIENT

Sign in for Period of Care 1 (0730-0815). From the Patient List, select Dorothy Grant in Room 201; however, do not go to the Nurses' Station yet.

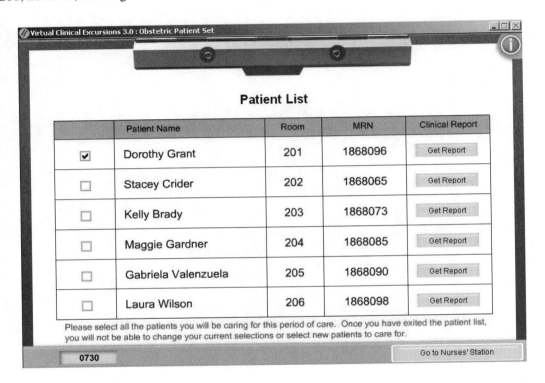

■ REPORT

In hospitals, when one shift ends and another begins, the outgoing nurse who attended a patient will give a verbal and sometimes a written summary of that patient's condition to the incoming nurse who will assume care for the patient. This summary is called a report and is an important source of data to provide an overview of a patient. Your first task is to get the clinical report on Dorothy Grant. To do this, click **Get Report** in the far right column in this patient's row. From a brief review of this summary, identify the problems and areas of concern that you will need to address for this patient.

When you have finished noting any areas of concern, click **Go to Nurses' Station**.

■ CHARTS

You can access Dorothy Grant's chart from the Nurses' Station or from the patient's room (201). From the Nurses' Station, click on the chart rack or on the **Chart** icon in the tool bar at the top of your screen. Next, click on the chart labeled **201** to open the medical record for Dorothy Grant. Click on the **Emergency Department** tab to view a record of why this patient was admitted.

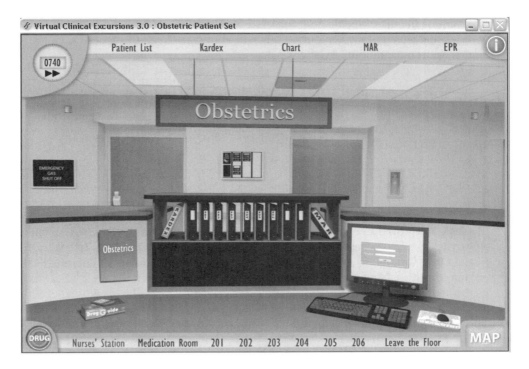

How many days has Dorothy Grant been in the hospital?

What tests were done upon her arrival in the Emergency Department and why?

What was the reason for her admission?

You should also click on **Surgical Reports** to learn whether any procedures were performed and when. Finally, review the **Nursing Admission** and **History and Physical** to learn about the health history of this patient. When you are done reviewing the chart, click **Return to Nurses' Station**.

■ MEDICATIONS

Open the Medication Administration Record (MAR) by clicking on the **MAR** icon in the tool bar at the top of your screen. *Remember:* The MAR automatically opens to the first occupied room number on the floor—which is not necessarily your patient's room number! Since you need to access Dorothy Grant's MAR, click on tab **201** (her room number). Always make sure you are giving the *Right Drug to the Right Patient!*

Examine the list of medications ordered for Dorothy Grant. In the table below, list the medications that need to be given during this period of care (0730-0815). For each medication, note the dosage, route, and time to be given.

Time	Medication	Dosage	Route

Click on **Return to Nurses' Station**. Next, click on **201** on the bottom tool bar and then verify that you are indeed in Dorothy Grant's room. Select **Clinical Alerts** (the icon to the right of Initial Observations) to check for any emerging data that might affect your medication administration priorities. Next, go to the patient's chart (click on the **Chart** icon; then click on **201**). When the chart opens, select the **Physician's Orders** tab.

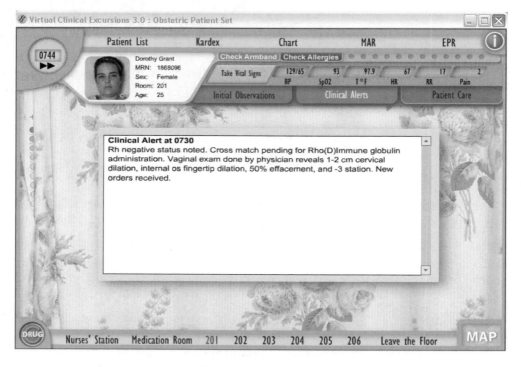

Review the orders. Have any new medications been ordered? Return to the MAR (click **Return to Room 201**; then click **MAR**). Verify that the new medications have been correctly transcribed to the MAR. Mistakes are sometimes made in the transcription process in the hospital setting, and it is sound practice to double-check any new order.

Are there any patient assessments you will need to perform before administering these medications? If so, return to Room 201 and click on **Patient Care** and then **Physical Assessment** to complete those assessments before proceeding.

Now click on the **Medication Room** icon in the tool bar at the bottom of your screen to locate and prepare the medications for Dorothy Grant.

In the Medication Room, you must access the medications for Dorothy Grant from the specific dispensing system in which each medication is stored. Locate each medication that needs to be given in this time period and click on **Put Medication on Tray** as appropriate. (*Hint:* Look in **Unit Dosage** drawer first.) When you are finished, click on **Close Drawer** and then on **View Medication Room**. Now click on the medication tray on the counter on the left side of the medication room screen to begin preparing the medications you have selected. (*Remember:* You can also click **Preparation** in the tool bar at the top of the screen.)

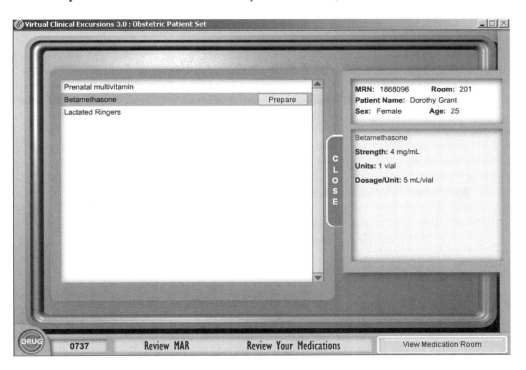

In the preparation area, you should see a list of the medications you put on the tray in the previous steps. Click on the first medication and then click **Prepare**. Follow the onscreen instructions of the Preparation Wizard, providing any data requested. As an example, let's follow the preparation process for betamethasone, one of the medications due to be administered to Dorothy Grant during this period of care. To begin, click on **Betamethasone**; then click **Prepare**. Now work through the Preparation Wizard sequence as detailed below:

Amount of medication in the ampule: 5 mL.
Enter the amount of medication you will draw up into a syringe: **3** mL.
Click **Next**.
Select the patient you wish to set aside the medication for: **Room 201, Dorothy Grant**.
Click **Finish**.
Click **Return to Medication Room**.

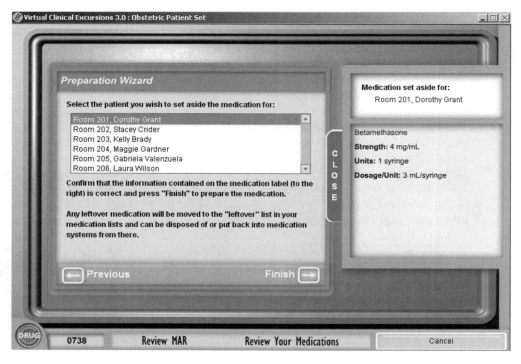

Follow this same basic process for the other medications due to be administered to Dorothy Grant during this period of care. (*Hint:* Look in **IV Storage** and **Automated System**.)

PREPARATION WIZARD EXCEPTIONS

- Some medications in *Virtual Clinical Excursions—Obstetrics* are prepared by the pharmacy (e.g., IV antibiotics) and taken to the patient room as a whole. This is common practice in most hospitals.
- Blood products are not administered by students through the *Virtual Clinical Excursions—Obstetrics* simulations since blood administration follows specific protocols not covered in this program.
- The *Virtual Clinical Excursions—Obstetrics* simulations do not allow for mixing more than one type of medication, such as regular and Lente insulins, in the same syringe. In the clinical setting, when multiple types of insulin are ordered for a patient, the regular insulin is drawn up first, followed by the longer-acting insulin. Insulin is always administered in a special unit-marked syringe.

Now return to Room 201 (click on **201** on the bottom tool bar) to administer Dorothy Grant's medications.

At any time during the medication administration process, you can perform a further review of systems, take vital signs, check information contained within the chart, or verify patient identity and allergies. Inside Dorothy Grant's room, click **Take Vital Signs**. (*Note:* These findings change over time to reflect the temporal changes you would find in a patient similar to Dorothy Grant.)

When you have gathered all the data you need, click on **Patient Care** and then select **Medication Administration**. Any medications you prepared in the previous steps should be listed on the left side of your screen. Let's continue the administration process with the betamethasone ordered for Dorothy Grant. Click to highlight **Betamethasone** in the list of medications. Next, click on the down arrow to the right of **Select** and choose **Administer** from the drop-down menu. This will activate the Administration Wizard. Complete the Wizard sequence as follows:

- Route: **Injection**
- Method: **Intramuscular**
- Site: **Any**
- Click **Administer to Patient** arrow.
- Would you like to document this administration in the MAR? **Yes**
- Click **Finish** arrow.

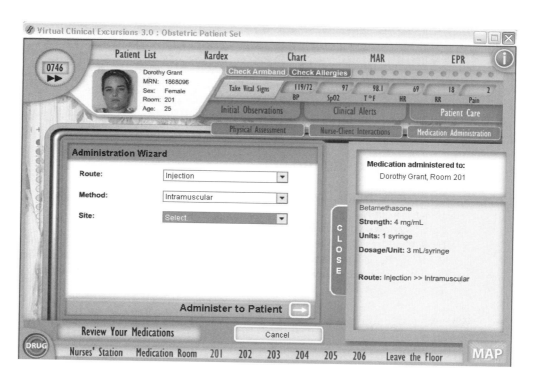

Your selections are recorded by a tracking system and evaluated on a Medication Scorecard stored under Preceptor's Evaluations. This scorecard can be viewed, printed, and given to your instructor. To access the Preceptor's Evaluations, click on **Leave the Floor**. When the Floor Menu appears, select **Look at Your Preceptor's Evaluation**. Then click on **Medication Scorecard** inside the box with Dorothy Grant's name (see example on the following page).

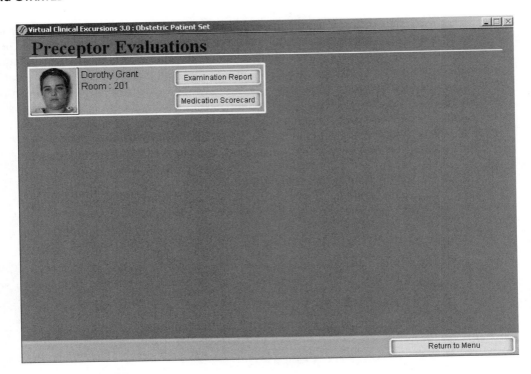

■ MEDICATION SCORECARD

- First, review Table A. Was betamethasone given correctly? Did you give the other medications as ordered?
- Table B shows you which (if any) medications you gave incorrectly.
- Table C addresses the resources used for Dorothy Grant. Did you access the patient's chart, MAR, EPR, or Kardex as needed to make safe medication administration decisions?
- Did you check the patient's armband to verify her identity? Did you check whether your patient had any known allergies to medications? Were vital signs taken?

When you have finished reviewing the scorecard, click **Return to Evaluations** and then **Return to Menu**.

■ VITAL SIGNS

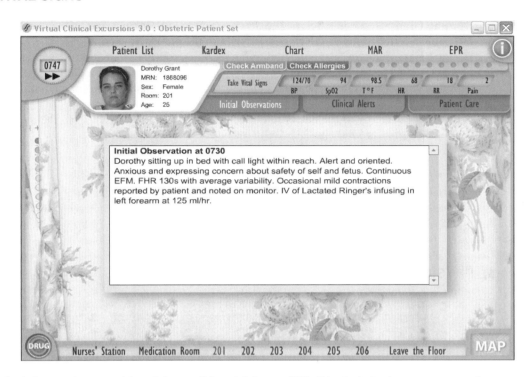

Vital signs, often considered the traditional "signs of life," include body temperature, heart rate, respiratory rate, blood pressure, oxygen saturation of the blood, and pain level.

Inside Dorothy Grant's room, click **Take Vital Signs**. (*Note:* If you are following this detailed tour step by step, you will need to **Restart the Program** from the Floor Menu, sign in again, and navigate to Room 201.) Collect vital signs for this patient and record them below. Note the time at which you collected each of these data. (*Remember:* You can take vital signs at any time. The data change over time to reflect the temporal changes you would find in a patient similar to Dorothy Grant.)

Vital Signs	Findings/Time
Blood pressure	
O$_2$ saturation	
Heart rate	
Respiratory rate	
Temperature	
Pain rating	

After you are done, click on the **EPR** icon located in the tool bar at the top of the screen. Your username and password are automatically provided. Click on **Login** to enter the EPR. To access Dorothy Grant's records, click on the down arrow next to Patient and choose her room number, **201**. Select **Vital Signs** as the category. Next, in the empty time column on the far right, record the vital signs data you just collected in the patient's room. (*Note:* If you need help with this process, see page 16.) Now compare these findings with the data you collected earlier for this patient's vital signs. Use these earlier findings to establish a baseline for each of the vital signs.

    a.   Are any of the data you collected significantly different from the baseline for a particular vital sign?

        Circle One: Yes   No

    b.   If "Yes," which data are different?

■ PHYSICAL ASSESSMENT

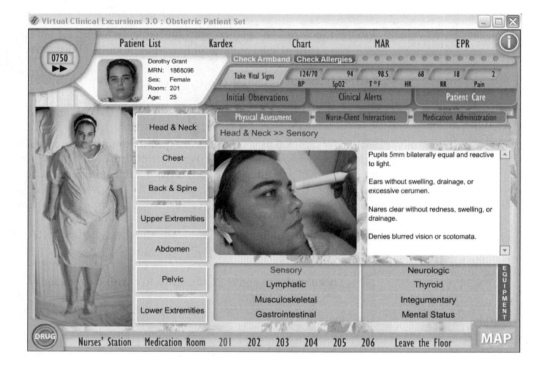

After you have finished examining the EPR for vital signs, click **Exit EPR** to return to Room 201. Click **Patient Care** and then **Physical Assessment**. Think about the information you received in the report at the beginning of this shift, as well as what you may have learned about this patient from the chart. Based on this, what area(s) of examination should you pay most attention to at this time? Is there any equipment you should be monitoring? Conduct a physical assessment of the body areas and systems that you consider priorities for Dorothy Grant. For example, select **Head & Neck**; then click on and assess **Sensory** and **Lymphatic**. Complete any other assessment(s) you think are necessary at this time. In the following table, record the data you collected during this examination.

Area of Examination	Findings
Head & Neck Sensory	
Head & Neck Lymphatic	

After you have finished collecting these data, return to the EPR. Compare the data that were already in the record with those you just collected.

    a. Are any of the data you collected significantly different from the baselines for this patient?

       Circle One: Yes   No

    b. If "Yes," which data are different?

■ NURSE-CLIENT INTERACTIONS

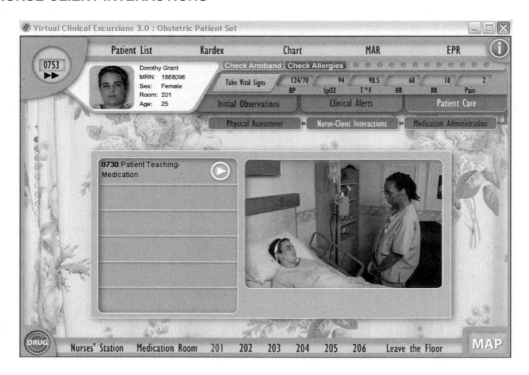

Click on **Patient Care** from inside Dorothy Grant's room (201). Now click on **Nurse-Client Interactions** to access a short video titled **Patient Teaching—Medication**, which is available for viewing at or after 0730 (based on the virtual clock in the upper left corner of your screen; see *Note* below). To begin the video, click on the white arrow next to its title. You will observe a nurse communicating with Dorothy Grant. There are many variations of nursing practice, some exemplifying "best" practice and some not. Note whether the nurse in this interaction displays professional behavior and compassionate care. Are her words congruent with what is going on with the patient? Does this interaction "feel right" to you? If not, how would you handle this situation differently? Explain.

Note: If the video you wish to view is not listed, this means you have not yet reached the correct virtual time to view that video. Check the virtual clock; you may return to access the video once its designated time has occurred—as long as you do so within the same period of care. Or you can click on the fast-forward icon within the virtual clock to advance the time by 2-minute intervals. You will then need to click again on **Patient Care** and **Nurse-Client Interactions** to refresh the screen.

At least one Nurse-Client Interactions video is available during each period of care. Viewing these videos can help you learn more about what is occurring with a patient at a certain time and also prompt you to discern between nurse communications that are ideal and those that need improvement. Compassionate care and the ability to communicate clearly are essential components of delivering quality nursing care, and it is during your clinical time that you will begin to refine these skills.

■ COLLECTING AND EVALUATING DATA

Each of the activities you perform in the Patient Care environment generates a significant amount of assessment data. Remember that after you collect data, you can record your findings in the EPR. You can also review the EPR, patient's chart, videos, and MAR at any time. You will get plenty of practice collecting and then evaluating data in context of the patient's course.

Now, here's an important question for you:

> Did the previous sequence of exercises provide the most efficient way to assess Dorothy Grant?

For example, you went to the patient's room to get vital signs, then back to the EPR to enter data and compare your findings with extant data. Next, you went back to the patient's room to do a physical examination, then again back to the EPR to enter and review data. If this back-and-forth process of data collection and recording seemed inefficient, remember the following:

- Plan all of your nursing activities to maximize efficiency, while at the same time optimizing the quality of patient care. (Think about what data you might need before performing certain tasks. For example, do you need to check a heart rate before administering a cardiac medication or check an IV site before starting an infusion?)

- You collect a tremendous amount of data when you work with a patient. Very few people can accurately remember all these data for more than a few minutes. Develop efficient assessment skills, and record data as soon as possible after collecting them.

- Assessment data are only the starting point for the nursing process.

Make a clear distinction between these first exercises and how you actually provide nursing care. These initial exercises were designed to involve you actively in the use of different software components. This workbook focuses on sensible practices for implementing the nursing process in ways that ensure the highest-quality care of patients.

Most important, remember that a human being changes through time, and that these changes include both the physical and psychosocial facets of a person as a living organism. Think about this for a moment. Some patients may change physically in a very short time (a patient with emerging myocardial infarction) or more slowly (a patient with a chronic illness). Patients' overall physical and psychosocial conditions may improve or deteriorate. They may have effective coping skills and familial support, or they may feel alone and full of despair. In fact, each individual is a complex mix of physical and psychosocial elements, and at least some of these elements usually change through time.

Thus it is crucial that you *DO NOT* think of the nursing process as a simple one-time, five-step procedure consisting of assessment, nursing diagnosis, planning, implementation, and evaluation. Rather, the nursing process should be utilized as a creative and systematic approach to delivering nursing care. Furthermore, because all living organisms are constantly changing, we must apply the nursing process over and over. Each time we follow the nursing process for an individual patient, we refine our understanding of that patient's physical and psychosocial conditions based on collection and analysis of many different types of data. *Virtual Clinical Excursions—Obstetrics* will help you develop both the creativity and the systematic approach needed to become a nurse who is equipped to deliver the highest-quality care to all patients.

REDUCING MEDICATION ERRORS

Earlier in this detailed tour, you learned the basic steps of medication preparation and administration. The following simulations will allow you to practice those skills further—with an increased emphasis on reducing medication errors by using the Medication Scorecard to evaluate your work.

Sign in to work at Pacific View Regional Hospital for Period of Care 1. (*Note:* If you are already working with another patient or during another period of care, click on **Leave the Floor** and then **Restart the Program**; then sign in.)

From the Patient List, select Dorothy Grant. Then click on **Go to Nurses' Station**. Complete the following steps to prepare and administer medications to Dorothy Grant.

- Click on **Medication Room**.

- Click on **MAR** and then on tab **201** to determine prn medications that have been ordered for Dorothy Grant. (*Note:* You may click on **Review MAR** at any time to verify the correct medication order. Always remember to check the patient name on the MAR to make sure you have the correct patient's record—you must click on the correct room number tab within the MAR.) Click on **Return to Medication Room** after reviewing the correct MAR.

- Click on **Unit Dosage** (or on the Unit Dosage cabinet); from the close-up view, click on drawer **201**.

- Select the medications you would like to administer. After each selection, click **Put Medication on Tray**. When you are finished selecting medications, click **Close Drawer** and then **View Medication Room**.

- Click **Automated System** (or on the Automated System unit itself). Click **Login**.

- On the next screen, specify the correct patient and drawer location.

- Select the medication you would like to administer and click **Put Medication on Tray**. Repeat this process if you wish to administer other medications from the Automated System.

- When you are finished, click **Close Drawer** and **View Medication Room**.

- From the Medication Room, click **Preparation** (or on the preparation tray).

- From the list of medications on your tray, highlight the correct medication to administer and click **Prepare**.

- This activates the Preparation Wizard. Supply any requested information; then click **Next**.

- Now select the correct patient to receive this medication and click **Finish**.

- Repeat the previous three steps until all medications that you want to administer are prepared.

- You can click on **Review Your Medications** and then on **Return to Medication Room** when ready. Once you are back in the Medication Room, go directly to Dorothy Grant's room by clicking on **201** at the bottom of the screen.

- Inside the patient's room, administer the medication, utilizing the five rights of medication administration. After you have collected the appropriate assessment data and are ready for administration, click **Patient Care** and then **Medication Administration**. Verify that the correct patient and medication(s) appear in the left-hand window. Highlight the first medication you wish to administer; then click the down arrow next to Select. From the drop-down menu, select **Administer** and complete the Administration Wizard by providing any information requested. When the Wizard stops asking for information, click **Administer to Patient**. Specify **Yes** when asked whether this administration should be recorded in the MAR. Finally, click **Finish**.

■ **SELF-EVALUATION**

Now let's see how you did during your medication administration!

- Click on **Leave the Floor** at the bottom of your screen. From the Floor Menu, select **Look at Your Preceptor's Evaluation**. Then click **Medication Scorecard**.

The following exercises will help you identify medication errors, investigate possible reasons for these errors, and reduce or prevent medication errors in the future.

1. Start by examining Table A. These are the medications you should have given to Dorothy Grant during this period of care. If each of the medications in Table A has a ✓ by it, then you made no errors. Congratulations!

If any medication has an X by it, then you made one or more medication errors.

Compare Tables A and B to determine which of the following types of errors you made: Wrong Dose, Wrong Route/Method/Site, or Wrong Time. Follow these steps:
   a. Find medications in Table A that were given incorrectly.
   b. Now see if those same medications are in Table B, which shows what you actually administered to Dorothy Grant.
   c. Comparing Tables A and B, match the Strength, Dose, Route/Method/Site, and Time for each medication you administered incorrectly.
   d. Then, using the form below, list the medications given incorrectly and mark the errors you made for each medication.

Medication	Strength	Dosage	Route	Method	Site	Time
	❏	❏	❏	❏	❏	❏
	❏	❏	❏	❏	❏	❏
	❏	❏	❏	❏	❏	❏
	❏	❏	❏	❏	❏	❏

2. To help you reduce future medication errors, consider the following list of possible reasons for errors.

- Did not check drug against MAR for correct patient, correct date, correct time, correct drug, and correct dose.
- Did not check drug dose against MAR three times.
- Did not open the unit dose package in the patient's room.
- Did not correctly identify the patient using two identifiers.
- Did not administer the drug on time.
- Did not verify patient allergies.
- Did not check the patient's current condition or vital sign parameters.
- Did not consider why the patient would be receiving this drug.
- Did not question why the drug was in the patient's drawer.
- Did not check the physician's order and/or check with the pharmacist when there was a question about the drug or dose.
- Did not verify that no adverse effects had occurred from a previous dose.

Based on the list of possibilities you just reviewed, determine how you made each error and record the reason in the form below:

Medication	Reason for Error

3. Look again at Table B. Are there medications listed that are not in Table A? If so, you gave a medication to Dorothy Grant that she should not have received. Complete the following exercises to help you understand how such an error might have been made.

   a. Perhaps you gave a medication that was on Dorothy Grant's MAR for this period of care, without recognizing that a change had occurred in the patient's condition, which should have caused you to reconsider. Review patient records as necessary and complete the following form:

Medication	Possible Reasons Not to Give This Medication

   b. Another possibility is that you gave Dorothy Grant a medication that should have been given at a different time. Check her MAR and complete the form below to determine whether you made a Wrong Time error:

Medication	Given to Dorothy Grant at What Time	Should Have Been Given at What Time

c. Maybe you gave another patient's medication to Dorothy Grant. In this case, you made a Wrong Patient error. Check the MARs of other patients and use the form below to determine whether you made this type of error:

Medication	Given to Dorothy Grant	Should Have Been Given to

4. The Medication Scorecard provides some other interesting sources of information. For example, if there is a medication selected for Dorothy Grant but it was not given to her, there will be an X by that medication in Table A, but it will not appear in Table B. In that case, you might have given this medication to some other patient, which is another type of Wrong Patient error. To investigate further, look at Table D, which lists the medications you gave to other patients. See whether you can find any medications ordered for Dorothy Grant that were given to another patient by mistake. However, before you make any decisions, be sure to cross-check the MAR for other patients because the same medication may have been ordered for multiple patients. Use the following form to record your findings:

Medication	Should Have Been Given to Dorothy Grant	Given by Mistake to

5. Now take some time to review the medication exercises you just completed. Use the form below to create an overall analysis of what you have learned. Once again, record each of the medication errors you made, including the type of each error. Then, for each error you made, indicate specifically what you would do differently to prevent this type of error from occurring again.

Medication	Type of Error	Error Prevention Tactic

Submit this form to your instructor if required as a graded assignment, or simply use these exercises to improve your understanding of medication errors and how to reduce them.

Name: _____   Date: _____

The following icons are used throughout this workbook to help you quickly identify particular activities and assignments:

 Indicates a reading assignment—tells you which textbook chapter(s) you should read before starting each lesson

 Indicates a writing activity

 Marks the beginning of an interactive CD-ROM activity—signals you to open or return to your *Virtual Clinical Excursions—Obstetrics* CD-ROM

 Indicates additional CD-ROM instructions

 Indicates questions and activities that require you to consult your textbook

 Indicates the approximate time required to complete an exercise

Assessment and Health Promotion

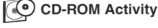 **Reading Assignment:** Assessment and Health Promotion (Chapter 5)

Patients: Maggie Gardner, Room 204
Gabriela Valenzuela, Room 205
Laura Wilson, Room 206

Goal: To identify the variations found in a pregnant patient's assessment, including health risk behaviors and health promotion techniques to assist in the optimal outcome for the fetus.

Objectives:

- Discuss the variations in a pregnant patient's assessment findings.
- Identify health risks in pregnant patients.
- Explore health promotion interventions that can and should be completed by the nurse caring for those patients with high-risk behaviors.

Exercise 1

 CD-ROM Activity

 20 minutes

Review pages 91-94 in your textbook to answer questions 1-3.

1. According to the textbook, what are the normal findings for a breast assessment?

• Sign in to work at Pacific View Regional Hospital on the Obstetrics Floor for Period of Care 1. (*Note*: If you are already in the virtual hospital from a previous exercise, click on **Leave the Floor** and then **Restart the Program** to get to the sign-in window.)
• From the Patient List, select Maggie Gardner.
• Click on **Go to Nurses' Station**.
• Go to the patient's room by clicking on **204** at the bottom of the screen.
• Click on the **Patient Care** icon.
• Click on the **Physical Assessment** tab.
• Click on **Chest** in the vertical row of yellow buttons.
• Click on the green button labeled **Breasts**. Review the breast assessment.

2. Compare and contrast the normal breast assessment findings described in the textbook with Maggie Gardner's findings.

 • Still in Maggie Gardner's room, click on **Chart** at the top of the screen.
• Click on chart **204**.
• Click on the **Nursing Admission** tab and review question 13 on page 5.

3. As a part of health promotion for this patient, complete the following:

a. Does Maggie Gardner do monthly breast self-exams?

b. Has she ever had a mammogram?

 c. According to the textbook, what is the recommendation regarding mammograms in Maggie Gardner's age group? (*Hint*: See Table 5-3 in your textbook.)

d. Based on your textbook reading, what should Maggie Gardner be taught about breast self-examination?

• According to the textbook, there are many barriers to seeking health care. We see this is true for Maggie Gardner. Continue reviewing the Nursing Admission section of her chart to answer the following questions regarding these barriers.

4. What are three barriers, identified on pages 100-101 of the textbook, to seeking health care?

5. Maggie Gardner, in her interaction with the nurse, identifies the barrier that prevented her from seeking heath care. What was this barrier?

Exercise 2

CD-ROM Activity

 40 minutes

 • Sign in to work at Pacific View Regional Hospital on the Obstetrics Floor for Period of Care 3. (*Note*: If you are already in the virtual hospital from a previous exercise, click on **Leave the Floor** and then **Restart the Program** to get to the sign-in window.)
• From the Patient List, select Laura Wilson.
• Click on **Go to Nurses' Station**.
• Click on **Chart** and then on **206**.
• Review the **History and Physical** and the **Nursing Admission** to obtain the following information.

Along with barriers to seeking and receiving health care, specific health risks occur during the childbearing years. In this exercise, we will consider these risks in relation to Laura Wilson in Room 206.

1. List the factors that put Laura Wilson at risk during her pregnancy.

2. In the Nursing Admission form, what does Laura Wilson verbalize about her use of drugs, tobacco, and alcohol in regard to her pregnancy and outcomes for her baby?

• Click on **Return to Nurses' Station**.
- Click on **206** at the bottom of the screen.
- Click on **Patient Care** and then **Nurse-Client Interactions**.
- Select and view the video titled **1530: Discharge Planning**. (*Note:* Check the virtual clock to see whether enough time has elapsed. You can use the fast-forward feature to advance the time by 2-minute intervals if the video is not yet available. Then click on **Patient Care** and **Nurse-Client Interactions** to refresh the screen.)
- After viewing the video, click on **Leave the Floor**.
- Click on **Restart the Program**.
- Sign in again to work at Pacific View Regional Hospital on the Obstetrics Floor, this time for Period of Care 4. (*Remember:* You are not able to visit patients or administer medications during Period of Care 4. You are able to review patients' records only.)
- From the Nurses' Station, click on **Chart** and then on **206**.
- Click on the **Consultations** tab and review the Psychiatric Consult.
- Next, click on **Nurse's Notes** and review.

Answer the following questions regarding your impression of the 1530 video interaction and your chart review.

3. What was the clinician's perspective of Laura Wilson and her current life situation?

4. What was your impression of Laura Wilson?

5. What does Laura Wilson say that indicates she may not understand HIV or is in denial that it is truly a medical concern?

6. From your review of the 1530 video and the Psychiatric Consult notes, what areas of health education (health promotion) need to be the focus for Laura Wilson?

Exercise 3

 CD-ROM Activity

 20 minutes

The head-to-toe assessment is a key part of obtaining data, both subjective and objective, from our patients. The following exercise will walk you through a head-to-toe assessment on a pregnant patient. The goal of this exercise is to identify areas in each body system that are abnormal and recognize those that are pregnancy-related changes.

- Sign in to work at Pacific View Regional Hospital on the Obstetrics Floor for Period of Care 2. *(Note:* If you are already in the virtual hospital from a previous exercise, click on **Leave the Floor** and then **Restart the Program** to get to the sign-in window.)
- From the Patient List, select Gabriela Valenzuela.
- Click on **Go to Nurses' Station** and then on **205** at the bottom of the screen.
- Click on **Patient Care** and then **Physical Assessment**.
- Begin your assessment by clicking on **Head & Neck** (from the list of yellow buttons) and then selecting each of the system subcategories (the green buttons) to obtain the findings for that area. Continue clicking on the yellow and green buttons as you record your findings in question 1.

1. Below and on the next page, record any abnormal findings and any changes related to pregnancy from your head-to-toe assessment of Gabriela Valenzuela.

   a. Head & Neck

   b. Chest

   c. Back & Spine

   d. Upper Extremities

e. Abdomen

f. Pelvic

g. Lower Extremities

2. Once the health assessment is complete, what is the nurse's responsibility to the patient on return visits?

3. List five areas in which a nurse needs to educate women to help them maintain a healthy life.

4. Pelvic exams are recommended _____ until women are _____ years old. They

   are to be started when a female _____.

5. Holli, a 65-year-old, comes to you and states that she hates going to doctors because they always seem to be males, but that she needs to have a physical because it has been "years." Based on your reading, how could you help Holli overcome the barriers that she has? Also, what information could you provide that would help her be prepared for the examination?

LESSON 3

Violence Against Women

 Reading Assignment: Violence Against Women (Chapter 6)

Patient: Dorothy Grant, Room 201

Goal: To identify patients at risk for intimate partner violence, interventions to assist those at risk, and ways to educate and empower those individuals toward healthy relationships.

Objectives:

- Discuss the statistics related to intimate partner violence (IPV).
- List characteristics of battered women.
- Explore the myths and facts regarding IPV.
- Identify the nurse's role in regard to the battered woman or those affected by IPV.

In this lesson you will explore the nurse's role in intimate partner violence and the battered patient.

Exercise 1

Writing Activity

 15 minutes

To answer the questions in this exercise, review the information on pages 125-129 of the textbook.

1. Match the statistics on the right to the descriptions of abuse on the left.

d _____ Percentage of men who are victims of IPV

   c _____ Percentage of women who are victims of IPV

b _____ Number of women murdered per day as a result of IPV 3

e _____ Estimated number of women who are victims of IPV annually

   f _____ The increased risk pregnant individuals have of experiencing IPV 3x

a _____ Goal of *Healthy People 2010* as it relates to IPV (the number they want to see IPV decreased to)

a. 4 per 1000 women per year

b. 3

c. 4%-8%

d. 4%

e. 7 million per year

f. 3 times normal

Historically, women have often been treated inhumanely. This continues even today. Based on information from the textbook, please select true or false for each of the following questions.

2. In ancient Roman times, women were provided fair and equal treatment in relation to acts of adultery and public drunkenness.
   a. True
   b. False

3. As late as 2002, women in some Middle-Eastern cultures could legally be stoned to death or raped as punishment.
   a. True
   b. False

4. Until the Nineteenth Century, abuse of one's wife was legal in the United States.
   a. True
   b. False

5. Mental illness can be blamed for the majority of violent acts against women.
   a. True
   b. False

6. Children who are abused are more likely to abuse as adults compared with children who have never been abused.
   a. True
   b. False

7. Violent episodes are greater among _____Unempl.____ and those with low-income jobs.

8. _____Nat. AM____ and ____Alask.____ women report the highest rates of IPV in the United States.
nat.

Exercise 2

 CD-ROM Activity

 45 minutes

- Sign in to work at Pacific View Regional Hospital on the Obstetrics Floor for Period of Care 1. (*Note*: If you are already in the virtual hospital from a previous exercise, click on **Leave the Floor** and then **Restart the Program** to get to the sign-in window.)
- From the Patient List, select Dorothy Grant.
- Click on **Go to Nurses' Station**.
- Click on **Chart**.
- Click on the chart for Room **201**.
- Click on the **Nursing Admission** tab.

In addition to reading about Dorothy Grant's perspective on the abusive relationship she has experienced, review the characteristics of battered women found on pages 130-133 in the textbook.

1. What is the reality of Dorothy Grant's situation? How does that correlate with the textbook reading?

   Violence escalates during preg.

 • Still in Dorothy Grant's chart, review the **History and Physical** and the **Nursing Admission** as needed to answer question 2.

2. According to the textbook, battered women have certain characteristics. For each characteristic listed below and on the next page, discuss how Dorothy Grant compares with the textbook descriptions. Base your answers on what you have learned about the patient so far in your chart review. (*Note:* You will return to this list to add follow-up findings after viewing the 0810 video interaction between Dorothy Grant and the nurse.)

Financially dependent

dep. husband sole provider.

Few resources/support systems *— N/A bc her*

family is support

Blame themselves for what has taken place

She thinks her preg is causing it

State that they are not "good enough"

Bonding occurs out of fear and helplessness

strong bond due to sanctity of marriage from church

Low self-esteem

poor eye contact + statements

History of domestic violence in their family

father abusive to mother

Strong nurturing, yielding personality

desires to keep husband happy

Tolerate control from others easily

- tries to keep kids quiet when husband around

Experience deliberate/repeated physical or sexual assault

forced to have sex - blunt ab trauma.

→ • Click on **Return to Nurses' Station**.
• Click on Room **201** at the bottom of the screen.
• Click on the **Patient Care** and then **Nurse-Client Interactions**. (*Note:* Take notes as you watch the following video.)
• Select and view the video titled **0810: Monitoring/Patient Support**. (*Note:* Check the virtual clock to see whether enough time has elapsed. You can use the fast-forward feature to advance the time by 2-minute intervals if the video is not yet available. Then click on **Patient Care** and **Nurse-Client Interactions** to refresh the screen.)

3. In the video interaction what does Dorothy Grant verbalize that she should do to help prevent the violence?

if she did more tried harder.

4. In the video, what are the patient's concerns at the moment?

care for child + baby, protect herself

5. Return to question 2 and review your answers, keeping in mind what you have learned through the 0810 nurse-client interaction. Would you change any of your answers based on this observation? If so, what would you add or change?

Exercise 3

 CD-ROM Activity

 10 minutes

- Sign in to work at Pacific View Regional Hospital on the Obstetrics Floor for Period of Care 3. (*Note*: If you are already in the virtual hospital from a previous exercise, click on **Leave the Floor** and then **Restart the Program** to get to the sign-in window.)
- From the Patient List, select Dorothy Grant.
- Click on **Go to Nurses' Station**.
- Click on **Chart**.
- Click on the chart for Room **201**.
- Click on **Consultations** and review the Psychiatric Consult and the Social Work Consult.

Review the information regarding the myths and facts about intimate partner violence on page 130 in the textbook. Based on that information and your review of Dorothy Grant's chart, answer the following:

1. Dorothy Grant stays in the relationship because of ___*fear*___ and ___*dep.*___ .
2. The percentage of women who are battered during pregnancy is *4-8%*

3. Based on the information provided, in what phase of the abuse cycle is Dorothy Grant?

phase II Battering

4. According to the consults, Dorothy Grant has several options. What are some of the options that the social worker and psychiatric health care provider can offer her or assist her with?

Shelter placement, education, restraining order

5. Battering often escalates or begins during pregnancy.
   (a) True
   b. False

6. Dorothy Grant's husband blames her for the pregnancy.
   a. True
   b. False

7. Dorothy Grant stays in the relationship because she likes to be beaten and deliberately provokes the attacks on occasion.
   a. True
   (b.) False

Exercise 4

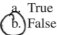 **CD-ROM Activity**

 10 minutes

- Sign in to work at Pacific View Regional Hospital on the Obstetrics Floor for Period of Care 4. (*Note*: If you are already in the virtual hospital from a previous exercise, click on **Leave the Floor** and then **Restart the Program** to get to the sign-in window.)
- From the Nurses' Station, click on **Kardex** and then on tab **201** to review Dorothy Grant's record. (*Remember:* You are not able to visit patients or administer medications during Period of Care 4. You are able to review patients' records only.)

1. What action was initiated on Wednesday to protect Dorothy Grant from her husband?

a security alert for him not to visit

2. What care plan diagnoses are appropriate for this patient's current life situation?

3. What other disciplines have been contacted or consulted that will ensure continuity of care for Dorothy Grant related to her abuse?

In your textbook, review pages 133-137 to assist in answering the following questions.

4. As a nurse caring for Dorothy Grant, what is your responsibility for reporting IPV?

5. What are the reporting requirements of the state in which you practice?

6. What are the resources available in your area for women who are experiencing intimate partner violence?

LESSON 4

Reproductive System Concerns, Contraception, and Infertility

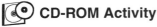 **Reading Assignment:** Reproductive Concerns (Chapter 7)
Contraception and Abortion (Chapter 9)
Infertility (Chapter 10)

Patients: Stacey Crider, Room 202
Kelly Brady, Room 203
Maggie Gardner, Room 204
Gabriela Valenzuela, Room 205
Laura Wilson, Room 206

Goal: Demonstrate an understanding of reproductive system concerns, contraception options, and infertility.

Objectives:

- Identify reproductive issues that can occur.
- Differentiate among the varying types of contraception available.
- Identify various methods of testing and treatment options for couples experiencing infertility.

Exercise 1

 CD-ROM Activity

 10 minutes

Review information on pages 145-146 in your textbook.

1. What is a normal length for a menstrual cycle?

2. What are the criteria required to diagnose an individual with amenorrhea?

• Sign in to work at Pacific View Regional Hospital on the Obstetrics Floor for Period of Care 1. (*Note*: If you are already in the virtual hospital from a previous exercise, click on **Leave the Floor** and then **Restart the Program** to get to the sign-in window.)

• From the Patient List, select Stacey Crider.

• Click on **Go to Nurses' Station**.

• Click on **Chart** and then on **202**.

• Click on **History and Physical**.

• Review the patient's gynecologic history. (*Hint:* See the bottom of page 1.)

3. Does Stacey Crider meet the textbook criteria for amenorrhea?

4. What is her history?

5. List three things that can cause amenorrhea.

Exercise 2

 CD-ROM Activity

 20 minutes

 Review pages 207-228 in the textbook.

1. What is contraception?

2. Providing contraception doesn't necessarily mean preventing _____.

 • Sign in to work at Pacific View Regional Hospital on the Obstetrics Floor for Period of Care 1. (*Note*: If you are already in the virtual hospital from a previous exercise, click on **Leave the Floor** and then **Restart the Program** to get to the sign-in window.)

• From the Patient List, select Kelly Brady, Gabriela Valezuela, and Laura Wilson.

• Click on **Go to Nurses' Station**.

• Click on **Chart** and then on **203** for Kelly Brady's chart.

• Review the **History and Physical**.

• Repeat the previous two steps for Gabriela Valenzuela and Laura Wilson.

3. Based on your review of their charts, list the birth control method each of these women were using prior to their current pregnancies.

Kelly Brady

Gabriela Valenzuela

Laura Wilson

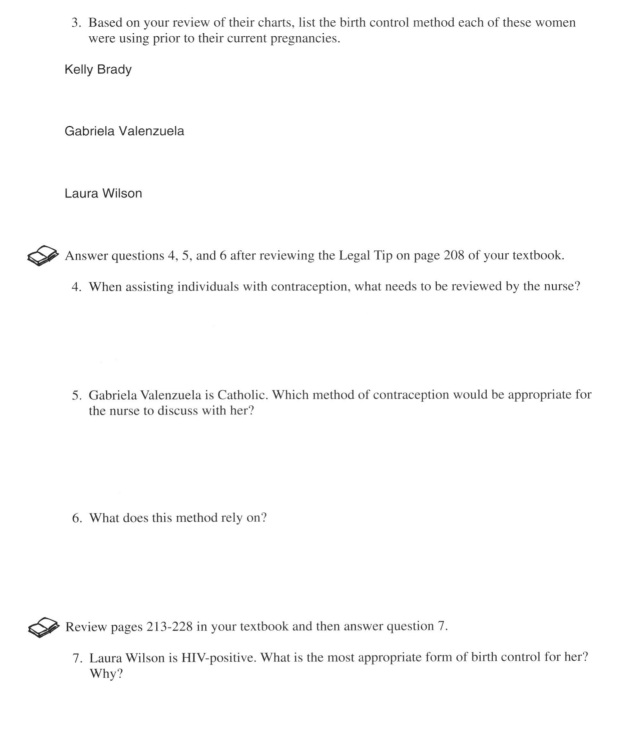 Answer questions 4, 5, and 6 after reviewing the Legal Tip on page 208 of your textbook.

4. When assisting individuals with contraception, what needs to be reviewed by the nurse?

5. Gabriela Valenzuela is Catholic. Which method of contraception would be appropriate for the nurse to discuss with her?

6. What does this method rely on?

Review pages 213-228 in your textbook and then answer question 7.

7. Laura Wilson is HIV-positive. What is the most appropriate form of birth control for her? Why?

Exercise 3

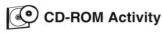 **CD-ROM Activity**

 20 minutes

 Review Chapter 10 in your textbook.

1. _____% of the reproductive age population has a problem with infertility.

2. At the age of _____ the incidence of infertility in women increases.

Maggie Gardner is 41 years old. Let's consider some of the options she had while attempting to get pregnant.

3. List two factors that affect female fertility.

4. List two factors that affect male fertility.

 • Sign in to work at Pacific View Regional Hospital on the Obstetrics Floor for Period of Care 1. (*Note*: If you are already in the virtual hospital from a previous exercise, click on **Leave the Floor** and then **Restart the Program** to get to the sign-in window.)
   • From the Patient List, select Maggie Gardner.
   • Click on **Go to Nurses' Station**.
   • Click on **Chart** and then on **204**.
   • Review the **History and Physical**.

5. Maggie Gardner was married _____ years prior to conceiving the first time.

6. Based on the textbook reading, which of the following would Maggie Gardner have been diagnosed with if she had chosen to get treatment after a year of attempting to get pregnant?

   a. Primary infertility
   b. Secondary infertility

Review pages 238-244 in your textbook to answer the following questions.

7. What four tests can be completed on a female patient to determine the causes of infertility?

8. What two tests can be completed on a male patient to determine the causes of infertility?

9. What test is used to assess a couple to determine adequacy of coital technique?

10. What methods are available to assist the infertile couple in conceiving?

11. What methods did Maggie Gardner and her husband use to assist in getting pregnant? (*Hint*: Review the OB history in the History and Physical.)

LESSON 5

Sexually Transmitted and Other Infections

 Reading Assignment: Sexually Transmitted and Other Infections (Chapter 8)

Patients: Stacey Crider, Room 202
Gabriela Valenzuela, Room 205
Laura Wilson, Room 206

Goal: Demonstrate an understanding of the identification and management of selected sexually transmitted and other infections in pregnant women.

Objectives:

- Assess and plan care for a pregnant woman with bacterial vaginosis.
- Explain the importance of prophylactic Group B streptococcus treatment.
- Identify risk factors for acquiring HIV infection.
- Prioritize information to be included in patient teaching related to HIV infection.

In this lesson you will assess and evaluate the care provided to three hospitalized pregnant women in regard to sexually transmitted infections (STIs).

Exercise 1

 CD-ROM Activity

15 minutes

- Sign in to work at Pacific View Regional Hospital on the Obstetrics Floor for Period of Care 1. (*Note*: If you are already in the virtual hospital from a previous exercise, click on **Leave the Floor** and then **Restart the Program** to get to the sign-in window.)
- From the Patient List, select Stacey Crider.
- Click on **Go to Nurses' Station**.
- Click on **Chart** and then on **202**.
- Click on **History and Physical**.

1. In the table below, describe Stacey Crider's vaginal discharge on admission. How does it compare with the description of bacterial vaginosis found on pages 194-195 in the textbook?

	Stacey Crider's Discharge	Textbook Description
Appearance		
Amount		
Odor		

2. Consult Table 8-4 on page 195 in the textbook. How is bacterial vaginosis diagnosed?

3. Consult Table 8-5 on page 196 in the textbook. Which medications are recommended for treating bacterial vaginosis during pregnancy?

➤ • Now click on **Physician's Orders** in the chart.
  • Scroll down to the admitting physician's orders on Tuesday at 0630.

4. What are Stacey Crider's admission diagnoses?

5. Explain how Stacey Crider's admission diagnoses are likely to be related.

6. Which medication did Stacey Crider's physician order to treat her bacterial vaginosis?

7. Assume that Stacey Crider is discharged home on day 4 of the prescribed treatment with the medication you identified in question 6. What specific information about this medication should she be taught? (*Hint*: Check page 195 in the textbook.)

Exercise 2

 CD-ROM Activity

15 minutes

- Sign in to work at Pacific View Regional Hospital on the Obstetrics Floor for Period of Care 1. (*Note*: If you are already in the virtual hospital from a previous exercise, click on **Leave the Floor** and then **Restart the Program** to get to the sign-in window.)
- From the Patient List, select Gabriela Valenzuela.
- Click on **Go to Nurses' Station**.
- Click on **Chart** and then on **205**.
- Click on **History and Physical** and scroll to the plan at the end of this document.

1. What is the medical plan of care for Gabriela Valenzuela?

2. Is Gabriela Valenzuela known to be positive for Group B streptococcus (GBS)?

Read about Group B streptococcus on pages 197-198 in your textbook; then answer questions 3 through 6.

3. List risk factors for neonatal GBS infection. Which risk factor applies to Gabriela Valenzuela?

4. Since pregnant women with GBS in the vagina are almost always asymptomatic, why does Gabriela Valenzuela need to be treated for this organism?

- Click on **Physician's Orders**.
- Scroll to the admission orders written Tuesday at 2100.

5. What medication/dosage/frequency will Gabriela Valenzuela receive for Group B strep pro-phylaxis?

6. How does this order compare with the treatment regimen recommended in your textbook?

Exercise 3

 CD-ROM Activity

 35 minutes

- Sign in to work at Pacific View Regional Hospital on the Obstetrics Floor for Period of Care 1. (*Note*: If you are already in the virtual hospital from a previous exercise, click on **Leave the Floor** and then **Restart the Program** to get to the sign-in window.)
- From the Patient List, select Laura Wilson.
- Click on **Go to Nurses' Station**.
- Click on **Chart** and then on **206**.
- Click on **Nursing Admission**.

1. What risk factors for acquiring an STI are identified on Laura Wilson's Nursing Admission form?

 2. List specific risk factors for acquiring HIV infection. (*Hint:* See page 191 in the textbook.) Underline the risk factors that are present in Laura Wilson's history.

3. What did the admitting nurse document about Laura Wilson's knowledge and acceptance of her HIV diagnosis?

 • Click on **Return to Nurses' Station**.
   • Click on **Patient Care** and then **Nurse-Client Interactions**.
   • Select and view the video titled **0800: Teaching—HIV in Pregnancy**. (*Note:* Check the virtual clock to see whether enough time has elapsed. You can use the fast-forward feature to advance the time by 2-minute intervals if the video is not yet available. Then click on **Patient Care** and **Nurse-Client Interactions** to refresh the screen.)

4. Does Laura Wilson appear to be fully aware of the implications of HIV infection? State the rationale for your answer.

5. What coping mechanism is Laura Wilson exhibiting in the video interaction?

 • Click on **Chart**.
   • Click on **Nursing Admission**.

6. Laura Wilson needs education on all of the following topics. Which would you choose to teach her about at this time?

   _____ Safer sex

   _____ Medication side effects and importance of compliance

   _____ Need for medical follow-up and medication for the baby

   _____ Impact of HIV on birth plans

7. Give a rationale for your answer to question 6.

Nursing Care During Pregnancy

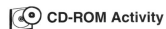 **Reading Assignment:** Nursing Care During Pregnancy (Chapter 16)

Patients: Kelly Brady, Room 203
Maggie Gardner, Room 204
Laura Wilson, Room 206

Goal: Demonstrate an understanding of the nursing care provided to women during normal pregnancy.

Objectives:

- Identify common physical and psychologic findings associated with each trimester of pregnancy.
- Describe differences in the normal pregnancy changes experienced by adolescent and older mothers.

In this lesson you will identify physical and psychologic pregnancy changes as they occur in three women at different gestational ages.

Exercise 1

 CD-ROM Activity

 20 minutes

Read the section on Diagnosis of Pregnancy on page 381 in your textbook.

1. List the subjective presumptive indicators of pregnancy identified in your textbook.

 • Sign in to work at Pacific View Regional Hospital on the Obstetrics Floor for Period of Care 1. (*Note*: If you are already in the virtual hospital from a previous exercise, click on **Leave the Floor** and then **Restart the Program** to get to the sign-in window.)
*   From the Patient List, select Maggie Gardner.
*   Click on **Go to Nurses' Station**.
*   Click on **Chart** and then **204**.
*   Click on **Nursing Admission**.

2. Place an X beside each of the subjective presumptive indicators of pregnancy that apply to Maggie Gardner according to the Nursing Admission.

    _____   Amenorrhea

    _____   Nausea/vomiting

    _____   Breast tenderness

    _____   Urinary frequency

    _____   Fatigue

    _____   Quickening

3. Uterine enlargement is considered a _____ indicator of pregnancy.

4. List three positive indicators of pregnancy.

 • Click on **Return to Nurses' Station**.
*   Click on Room **204** at the bottom of the screen.
*   Click on **Patient Care** and then **Physical Assessment**.
*   Perform a focused physical assessment by clicking on **Abdomen** and then on **Reproductive**.

5. What probable and positive pregnancy indicators are found in the abdominal assessment?

Probable

Positive

📖 Read the section on Estimating Date of Birth on page 381 in your textbook.

➡ • Click on **Chart** and then on **204**.
   • Click on **Nursing Admission**.
   • Scroll to the Pregnancy section on page 5.

6. What is recorded as Maggie Gardner's LMP?

7. Using Nagele's Rule, calculate Maggie Gardner's EDB. Explain how you calculated this date.

Exercise 2

💿 **CD-ROM Activity**

🕐 20 minutes

📖 Laura Wilson and Kelly Brady represent age extremes among women of childbearing age. Read the section on Adolescent Pregnancy on pages 422-423 in your textbook.

1. About 1 million adolescents in the United States, or _____ of every _____ girls, become

   pregnant each year. Most of the pregnancies are _____. _____% of these

   pregnancies end in induced abortion. _____ adolescents currently have the

   highest birth rate, although the rate for _____ is also high. Of girls who become

   pregnant, _____% are repeat pregnancies.

2. List common characteristics of pregnant adolescents, according to your textbook.

 • Sign in to work at Pacific View Regional Hospital on the Obstetrics Floor for Period of Care 4. (*Note*: If you are already in the virtual hospital from a previous exercise, click on **Leave the Floor** and then **Restart the Program** to get to the sign-in window.)
• Click on **Chart** and then on **206** for Laura Wilson's chart. (*Remember:* You are not able to visit patients or administer medications during Period of Care 4. You are able to review patients' records only.)
• Click on **Nursing Admission**.

3. Based on your chart review, how does Laura Wilson compare with the textbook profile of the pregnant adolescent? Explain how each of the characteristics you listed in question 2 applies (or does not apply) to Laura Wilson.

 Read the section on Women Older Than 35 Years on page 424 in your textbook.

4. List common characteristics of older primiparous women according to your textbook.

 • Click on **Return to Nurses' Station**.
• Click on **Chart** and then on **203** for Kelly Brady's chart.
• Click on **Nursing Admission**.

5. Based on your chart review, how does Kelly Brady compare with the textbook profile of the older primiparous woman? Explain how each of the characteristics you listed in question 4 applies (or does not apply) to Kelly Brady.

6. Women 35 years and older are more likely than younger primiparas to have

_____ infants, _____, and _____.

Exercise 3

CD-ROM Activity

15 minutes

- Sign in to work at Pacific View Regional Hospital on the Obstetrics Floor for Period of Care 4. (*Note*: If you are already in the virtual hospital from a previous exercise, click on **Leave the Floor** and then **Restart the Program** to get to the sign-in window.)
- Click on **Chart** and then on **204** for Maggie Gardner's chart. (*Remember:* You are not able to visit patients or administer medications during Period of Care 4. You are able to review patients' records only.)
- Click on **Nursing Admission**.

1. What is Maggie Gardner's gestational age?

2. Maggie Gardner is in the _____ trimester of pregnancy.

→ - Click on **Return to Nurses' Station**.
- Click on **Chart** and then on **206** for Laura Wilson's chart.
- Click on **Nursing Admission**.

3. What is Laura Wilson's gestational age?

4. Laura Wilson is in the _____ trimester of pregnancy.

Read the section on Adaptation to Pregnancy on pages 381-388 in your textbook.

5. Match each of the following behaviors in the pregnant woman with the trimester of pregnancy in which it is most likely to occur.

_____ Has fantasies about the fetus

_____ Is more interested in relationships with her mother and other women who are or have been pregnant

_____ Demonstrates emotional lability

_____ Ready for the pregnancy to end

_____ Has ambivalent feelings

_____ May experience increased desire for sex because of increased pelvic congestion

_____ Realistically prepares for birth and parenting the child

a. Second trimester

b. Third trimester

c. Throughout pregnancy

LESSON **8**

Nursing Care During Labor and Birth

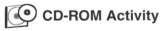 **Reading Assignment:** Nursing Care During Labor (Chapter 21)

Patients: Dorothy Grant, Room 201
Gabriela Valenzuela, Room 205
Laura Wilson, Room 206

Goal: Demonstrate an understanding of the normal labor and birth process.

Objectives:

- Assess and identify signs and symptoms present in each phase of Stage I labor.
- Describe appropriate nursing care for the patient in Stage I labor.

In this lesson you will plan and evaluate care for three patients in Stage I labor.

Exercise 1

 CD-ROM Activity

20 minutes

- Sign in to work at Pacific View Regional Hospital on the Obstetrics Floor for Period of Care 1. (*Note*: If you are already in the virtual hospital from a previous exercise, click on **Leave the Floor** and then **Restart the Program** to get to the sign-in window.)
- From the Patient List, select Dorothy Grant.
- Click on **Go to Nurses' Station**.
- Click on **Chart** and then on **201**.
- Click on **Nurse's Notes**.
- Scroll to the entry for 0730.

1. List the findings from Dorothy Grant's most recent cervical exam.

• Click on **Return to Nurses' Station**.
- Click on **EPR**.
- Click **Login**.
- Select **201** as the patient's room and **Obstetrics** as the category.

2. At 0700, what was the recorded frequency and duration of Dorothy Grant's contractions?

 • Now select **Vital Signs** as the category.

3. At 0700, what was Dorothy Grant's recorded pain level?

 Consult Table 21-3 on page 531 in your textbook.

4. At this time, which phase of Stage I labor is Dorothy Grant in?

5. For each specific assessment listed below, compare the typical findings for latent labor with Dorothy Grant's current condition.

Assessment	Typical Findings for Latent Labor	Findings for Dorothy Grant
Cervical dilation		
Contraction frequency		
Contraction duration		
Contraction strength		

6. List the typical behaviors in latent phase labor.

• Click on **Exit EPR**.
 • Click on **201** at the bottom of the screen.
 • Click on **Patient Care** and then **Nurse-Client Interactions**.
 • Select and view the video titled **0810: Monitoring/Patient Support**. (*Note:* Check the virtual clock to see whether enough time has elapsed. You can use the fast-forward feature to advance the time by 2-minute intervals if the video is not yet available. Then click on **Patient Care** and **Nurse-Client Interactions** to refresh the screen.)

7. Based on the video interaction, place an X next to each characteristic that is true of Dorothy Grant.

   _____ Excited

   _____ Thoughts center on self, labor, and baby

   _____ Some apprehension

   _____ Pain fairly well controlled

   _____ Alert

   _____ Follows directions readily

   _____ Open to instructions

Exercise 2

 CD-ROM Activity

 45 minutes

 • Sign in to work at Pacific View Regional Hospital on the Obstetrics Floor for Period of Care 2. (*Note*: If you are already in the virtual hospital from a previous exercise, click on **Leave the Floor** and then **Restart the Program** to get to the sign-in window.)
 • From the Patient List, select Gabriela Valenzuela.

 Read the sections on Physical Nursing Care During Labor and Supportive Care During Labor and Birth, pages 541-551 in your textbook.

 • Click on **Go to Nurses' Station**.
 • Click on **Chart** and then on **205**.
 • Click on **Nurse's Notes**.
 • Scroll back to the entry for 0800.

1. What was Gabriela Valenzuela's condition at this time? What phase of labor was she experiencing?

Consult Table 21-1 on page 526 in your textbook.

2. As Gabriela Valenzuela progresses in labor, which phase will she enter next?

3. List the common interventions for active phase labor.

→ • Still in the Nurse's Notes, scroll to the entry for 1140.

4. How is Gabriela Valenzuela tolerating labor at this time? Do you believe she has entered active phase?

5. How could you determine for certain which phase of labor Gabriela Valenzuela is currently experiencing?

→ • Click on **Return to Nurses' Station**.
  • Click on **205** at the bottom of the screen.
  • Click on **Patient Care** and then **Nurse-Client Interactions**.
  • Select and view the video titled: **1140: Intervention—Bleeding, Comfort**. (*Note:* Check the virtual clock to see whether enough time has elapsed. You can use the fast-forward feature to advance the time by 2-minute intervals if the video is not yet available. Then click on **Patient Care** and **Nurse-Client Interactions** to refresh the screen.)

6. Based on the video interaction, place an X next to each intervention suggested or implemented by the nurse.

_____ Limit assessment techniques to between contractions

_____ Assist patient to cope with contractions

_____ Encourage patient to help her maintain breathing techniques

_____ Use comfort measures

_____ Encourage voluntary muscle relaxation and use of effleurage

_____ Apply counterpressure to sacrococcygeal area

_____ Offer encouragement and praise

_____ Keep patient aware of progress

_____ Offer analgesics as ordered

_____ Check bladder; encourage voiding

_____ Give oral care; offer fluids, food, ice chips as ordered

• Click on **Patient Care** and then **Nurse-Client Interactions**.
• Select and view the video titled **1155: Evaluation—Comfort Measures**. (*Note:* Check the virtual clock to see whether enough time has elapsed. You can use the fast-forward feature to advance the time by 2-minute intervals if the video is not yet available. Then click on **Patient Care** and **Nurse-Client Interactions** to refresh the screen.)

7. Based on the video interaction, place an X next to each intervention suggested or implemented by the nurse and/or Gabriela Valenzuela's husband.

_____ Limit assessment techniques to between contractions

_____ Assist patient to cope with contractions

_____ Encourage patient to help her maintain breathing techniques

_____ Use comfort measures

_____ Assist with position changes

_____ Encourage voluntary muscle relaxation and use of effleurage

_____ Apply counterpressure to sacrococcygeal area

_____ Offer encouragement and praise

_____ Keep patient aware of progress

_____ Offer analgesics as ordered

_____ Check bladder; encourage voiding

_____ Give oral care; offer fluids, food, ice chips as ordered

Exercise 3

 CD-ROM Activity

 30 minutes

Let's jump ahead to Period of Care 4. Remember, you are not able to visit patients during this shift, but you have access to all patient records. First, we'll review Dorothy Grant's status.

• Sign in to work at Pacific View Regional Hospital on the Obstetrics Floor for Period of Care 4. (*Note*: If you are already in the virtual hospital from a previous exercise, click on **Leave the Floor** and then **Restart the Program** to get to the sign-in window.)

• From the Nurses' Station, click on **EPR** and then on **Login**.

• Select **201** as the patient's room and **Obstetrics** as the category.

• Scroll to review the entries for Wednesday 1800 and 1815.

1. What are the findings from Dorothy Grant's cervical exam at 1815?

 Consult Table 21-3 on page 531 in your textbook.

2. At this time, which phase of Stage I labor is Dorothy Grant experiencing?

3. Complete the table below, listing typical findings for each assessment in the transition phase of Stage I labor.

Assessment	Typical Findings
Cervical dilation	
Contraction frequency	
Contraction duration	
Contraction strength	

4. List the typical behaviors seen in patients experiencing the transition phase of labor.

- Click on **Exit EPR**.
- Click on **Chart** and then on **201** for Dorothy Grant's chart.
- Click on **Nurse's Notes**.
- Read the notes recorded at 1800, 1815, and 1830 on Wednesday.

5. Based on information recorded in the EPR and Nurse's Notes, place an X next to each behavior Dorothy Grant exhibited during the transition phase of labor.

_____ Severe pain

_____ Frustration; fear of loss of control

_____ Writhing with contractions

_____ Nausea/vomiting

_____ Perspiration

_____ Shaking or tremors

_____ Feeling the need to defecate

Now let's review Laura Wilson's status.

- Click on **Return to Nurses' Station**.
- Click on **EPR** and then on **Login**.
- Select **206** as the patient's room and **Vital Signs** as the category.

6. Below, record Laura Wilson's assessment findings from 1815 on Wednesday.

Pain location

Pain intensity

- Now select **Obstetrics** as the category.

7. Below, record Laura Wilson's 1830 assessment findings.

Contraction frequency

Contraction duration

- Scroll back through earlier Obstetrics entries until you locate the results of Laura Wilson's most recent cervical exam.

8. When was Laura Wilson's most recent cervical examination performed? What were the results?

→ • Click on **Exit EPR**.
  • Click on **Chart** and then on **206** for Laura Wilson's chart.
  • Click **Nurse's Notes**.
  • Scroll to the note for Wednesday 1830.

9. According to this note, what event occurred at 1815?

 Read the information on Assessment of Amniotic Membranes and Fluid on pages 538-540 in your textbook. Also read the Procedure box on Tests for Rupture of Membranes on page 524.

10. List the immediate nursing actions appropriate for the situation you identified in question 9.

11. According to the Nurse's Notes and your textbook recommendations, did Laura Wilson's nurse handle this situation appropriately? Explain.

12. Based only on the information you have learned about Laura Wilson during this exercise, write the nursing diagnosis that you consider to be of highest priority for her at this time.

13. List several nursing interventions for the nursing diagnosis you wrote in question 12.

LESSON 9

Management of Discomfort

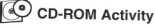 **Reading Assignment:** Management of Discomfort (Chapter 19)

Patients: Kelly Brady, Room 203
Gabriela Valenzuela, Room 205
Laura Wilson, Room 206

Goal: Demonstrate an understanding of the normal labor and birth process.

Objectives:

- Assess and identify factors that influence pain perception.
- Describe selected nonpharmacologic and pharmacologic measures for pain management during labor and birth.

In this lesson you will compare and contrast the pain management strategies used with three patients during labor and birth.

Exercise 1

 CD-ROM Activity

45 minutes

- Sign in to work at Pacific View Regional Hospital on the Obstetrics Floor for Period of Care 1. (*Note*: If you are already in the virtual hospital from a previous exercise, click on **Leave the Floor** and then **Restart the Program** to get to the sign-in window.)
- From the Patient List, select Laura Wilson.
- Click on **Get Report**.

1. What is Laura Wilson's condition when you assume care for her, according to the change-of-shift report?

• Click on **Go to Nurses' Station**.
• Click on Room **206** at the bottom of the screen.
• Read the **Initial Observations**.

2. What is your impression of Laura Wilson's condition?

 • Click on **Patient Care** and then **Nurse-Client Interactions**.
• Select and view the video titled **0730: Patient Assessment**. (*Note:* Check the virtual clock to see whether enough time has elapsed. You can use the fast-forward feature to advance the time by 2-minute intervals if the video is not yet available. Then click on **Patient Care** and **Nurse-Client Interactions** to refresh the screen.)

3. What is Laura Wilson's assessment of her current condition? How does this compare with the information you received from the shift report and the Initial Observations summary?

• Click on **Chart** and then on **206**.
• Click on **Nursing Admission**.

4. List Laura Wilson's admission diagnoses. (*Hint:* See page 1 of the Nursing Admission form.)

5. What is your perception of Laura Wilson's behavior? What data did you collect during this exercise that led you to this perception?

6. Think about the following questions and then discuss your ideas with your classmates: Do your personal values and beliefs contribute to your perception of Laura Wilson's behavior? If so, how? What nursing interventions might help to overcome your personal biases when dealing with Laura Wilson?

 Read the section on Factors Influencing Pain Response on pages 469-471 in your textbook.

 Continue reviewing Laura Wilson's **Nursing Admission** form as needed to answer question 7.

7. Each woman's pain during childbirth is unique and is influenced by a variety of factors. For each factor listed below, explain how that factor influences pain perception (in the middle column). Then, in the right column, list data from Laura Wilson's Nursing Admission that support how that factor might relate to her particular pain perception.

Factor	Typical Effect on Pain Perception	Laura Wilson's Supporting Data
Anxiety		
Previous experience		
Childbirth preparation		
Support		

Exercise 2

 CD-ROM Activity

 45 minutes

- Sign in to work at Pacific View Regional Hospital on the Obstetrics Floor for Period of Care 2. (*Note*: If you are already in the virtual hospital from a previous exercise, click on **Leave the Floor** and then **Restart the Program** to get to the sign-in window.)
- From the Patient List, select Gabriela Valenzuela.

Read the sections on Relaxing and Breathing Techniques (pages 471-473), Touch and Massage (page 476), and Systemic Analgesia (pages 478-481) in your textbook.

1. Focusing and relaxation techniques allow a woman in labor to rest and conserve energy by

   _____. While focusing on an object during a contraction, the

   woman _____ to reduce her _____.

   Varying breathing techniques are used to provide _____. All patterns begin and

   end with a _____.

2. Touch can communicate _____, _____, and _____.

   When using touch, it is important to determine the _____.

   Head, hand, back, and foot massage may be very effective in

   _____ and _____.

→ • Click on **Get Report**.

3. Is Gabriela Valenzuela in labor at this time? Give a rationale for your answer.

→ • Click **Go to Nurses' Station**.
- Click on Room **205** at the bottom of the screen.
- Click on **Patient Care** and then **Nurse-Client Interactions**.
- Select and view the video titled **1140: Intervention—Bleeding, Comfort**. (*Note:* Check the virtual clock to see whether enough time has elapsed. You can use the fast-forward feature to advance the time by 2-minute intervals if the video is not yet available. Then click on **Patient Care** and **Nurse-Client Interactions** to refresh the screen.)
- Click on **Chart**.
- Click on **Nurse's Notes**.
- Scroll to the entry for 1140 on Wednesday.

4. How is Gabriela Valenzuela tolerating labor at this time?

5. What pain interventions does the nurse implement at this time?

 Read the Medication Guide on fentanyl on page 480 in your textbook.

6. What is the action of this drug?

Let's begin the process for preparing and administering Gabriela Valenzuela's fentanyl dose.

- First, click on **Medication Room**.
- Next, click on **MAR** and then on tab **205**.
- Scroll down to the PRN Medication Administration Record for Wednesday.

7. What is the ordered dose of fentanyl?

- Click on **Return to Room 205**.
- Click on **Medication Room**.
- Click on **Automated System**.
- Click on **Login**.
- In box 1, click on **Gabriela Valenzuela, 205**.
- In box 2, click on **Automated System Drawer A-F**.
- Click on **Fentanyl citrate** and then **Put Medication on Tray**.
- Click on **Close Drawer** and then **View Medication Room**.
- Click on **Preparation**.
- Click on **Prepare** and follow the Preparation Wizard prompts to complete preparation of Gabriela Valenzuela's fentanyl dose. When the Wizard stops requesting information, click **Finish**.
- Click on **Return to Medication Room**.
- Click on **205** to go to the patient's room.

8. What additional assessments must be completed before you give Gabriela Valenzuela's medication?

9. Why is it important to check Gabriela Valenzuela's respirations prior to giving the dose of fentanyl?

10. What safety precautions should be in effect for Gabriela Valenzuela after she receives this dose of fentanyl?

→ • Click on **Patient Care** and then **Medication Administration**.
   • Click on **Review Your Medications** and verify the accuracy of your preparation. Click **Return to Room 205**.
   • Next, click the down arrow next to **Select** and choose **Administer**.
   • Follow the Administration Wizard prompts to administer Gabriela Valenzuela's fentanyl dose. (*Note:* Click **Yes** when asked whether to document this administration in the MAR.)
   • When the Wizard stops asking questions, click **Finish**.
   • Click on **Patient Care** and then **Nurse-Client Interactions**.
   • Select and view the video titled: **1155: Evaluation—Comfort Measures**. (*Note:* Check the virtual clock to see whether enough time has elapsed. You can use the fast-forward feature to advance the time by 2-minute intervals if the video is not yet available. Then click on **Patient Care** and **Nurse-Client Interactions** to refresh the screen.)

11. How effective were the interventions you identified in question 5?

12. Gabriela Valenzuela is experiencing _____. _____ is responsible for the dizziness as well as other side effects, including

_____, _____, and

_____.

13. What interventions does the nurse suggest to deal with this problem? List other interventions described in your textbook.

 At the end of the 1155 video, Gabriela Valenzuela states that she "doesn't want any needles" in her back. Read the section on Epidural Anesthesia or Analgesia (Block) on pages 485-488 in your textbook.

14. What could you tell Gabriela Valenzuela to help her make an informed decision about anesthesia for labor? Below, list advantages and disadvantages of epidural anesthesia.

Advantages	Disadvantages

Before leaving this period of care, let's see how you did preparing and administering the patient's medication.

- Click on **Leave the Floor**.
- Click on **Look at Your Preceptor's Evaluation**.
- Click on **Medication Scorecard** and review the evaluation. How did you do? (*Hint:* For a quick refresher on reading your Medication Scorecard, see page 22 in the **Getting Started** section of this workbook. For a more detailed tour on preparing and administering medications and interpreting your Scorecard, see pages 26-31 and 36-40.)

Exercise 3

 CD-ROM Activity

 20 minutes

 Read the section on General Anesthesia on pages 488-489 in your textbook.

- Sign in to work at Pacific View Regional Hospital on the Obstetrics Floor for Period of Care 4. (*Note*: If you are already in the virtual hospital from a previous exercise, click on **Leave the Floor** and then **Restart the Program** to get to the sign-in window.)
- From the Nurses' Station, click on **Chart** and then on **203** for Kelly Brady's chart. (*Remember:* You are not able to visit patients or administer medications during Period of Care 4. You are able to review patients' records only.)
- Click on **Nurse's Notes**.
- Scroll to the entry for 1730 on Wednesday.

 1. Why does the anesthesiologist plan to use general anesthesia during Kelly Brady's cesarean birth? (*Hint*: Read the section on Contraindications to Subarachnoid and Epidural Blocks on page 488 in your textbook.)

2. Why is Kelly Brady upset about receiving general anesthesia for her surgery?

- Click on **Physician's Orders**.
- Review the entry for Wednesday at 1540.

3. What preoperative medications are ordered for Kelly Brady?

- Click on **Return to Nurses' Station**.
- Click on the **Drug** icon in the lower left corner of your screen to access the Drug Guide.
- Use the Search box or the scroll bar to read about each of the drugs you listed in question 3.

4. All of these medications are given preoperatively to help prevent aspiration pneumonia. Using information from the Drug Guide and from the section on General Anesthesia in your textbook, match each of the medications below with the description of how it specifically works to prevent aspiration pneumonia.

_____ Sodium citrate/citric acid (Bicitra)

_____ Metoclopramide (Reglan)

_____ Ranitidine (Zantac)

a. Decreases the production of gastric acid

b. Prevents nausea and vomiting and accelerates gastric emptying

c. Neutralizes acidic stomach contents

5. During general anesthesia, a short-acting barbiturate or Ketamine is administered to

_____. A muscle relaxer is then given to

_____. A low concentration of a volatile halogenated agent

may be administered to _____.

6. How would you expect general anesthesia to affect Kelly Brady's baby? Why?

LESSON **10** ——————————————

Hypertensive Disorders in Pregnancy

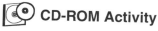 **Reading Assignment:** Hypertensive Disorders in Pregnancy (Chapter 30)

Patient: Kelly Brady, Room 203

Goal: Demonstrate an understanding of the identification and management of selected hypertensive complications of pregnancy.

Objectives:

- Assess and identify signs and symptoms present in the patient with severe preeclampsia.
- Explain how common signs and symptoms present in the patient with severe preeclampsia relate to the underlying pathophysiology of this disease.
- Identify the patient who has developed HELLP syndrome.
- Describe routine nursing care for the patient with severe preeclampsia who is receiving magnesium sulfate.

In this lesson you will assess and plan care for a patient with severe preeclampsia who then develops HELLP syndrome and delivers at 26 2/7 weeks gestation.

Exercise 1

 CD-ROM Activity

20 minutes

- Sign in to work at Pacific View Regional Hospital on the Obstetrics Floor for Period of Care 3. (*Note*: If you are already in the virtual hospital from a previous exercise, click on **Leave the Floor** and then **Restart the Program** to get to the sign-in window.)
- From the Patient List, select Kelly Brady.
- Click on **Go to Nurses' Station**.
- Click on **Chart** and then on **203**.
- Click on **History and Physical**.

1. What was Kelly Brady's admission diagnosis?

 2. Use the History and Physical and pages 785-786 in your textbook to complete the table below.

Sign/Symptom	Mild Preeclampsia	Severe Preeclampsia	Kelly Brady on Admission
Blood pressure			
Proteinuria			
Headache			
Reflexes			
Visual problems			
Epigastric pain			

→ • Click on **Physician's Orders** and find the admitting physician's orders on Tuesday at 1030.

3. What tests/procedures did Kelly Brady's physician order to confirm the diagnosis of severe preeclampsia?

→ • Click on **Physician's Notes**.
  • Scroll to the note for Wednesday 0730.

4. What subjective and objective data are recorded here that would support the diagnosis of severe preeclampsia?

Kelly Brady's 24-hour urine collection was completed and sent to the lab at 1230.

 • Click on **Laboratory Reports**.
• Scroll to find the Wednesday 1230 results.

5. Below, record the results of Kelly Brady's 24-hour urine collection.

6. Now list all the data you have collected during this exercise that confirm Kelly Brady's diagnosis of severe preeclampsia.

Exercise 2

 CD-ROM Activity

 20 minutes

• Sign in to work at Pacific View Regional Hospital on the Obstetrics Floor for Period of Care 1. (*Note*: If you are already in the virtual hospital from a previous exercise, click on **Leave the Floor** and then **Restart the Program** to get to the sign-in window.)
• From the Patient List, select Kelly Brady.
• Click on **Go to Nurses' Station**.
• Click on **203** at the bottom of the screen.
• Click on **Take Vital Signs**.

1. Record Kelly Brady's vital signs for 0730 below.

 • Click on **Patient Care** and then **Physical Assessment**.
• Select the various body areas (yellow buttons) and system subcategories (green buttons) as listed in question 2.

2. Record your findings from the focused assessment of Kelly Brady in the table below.

Assessment Area	Kelly Brady's Findings
Head & Neck Sensory	
Neurologic	
Chest Respiratory	
Abdomen Gastrointestinal	
Lower Extremities Neurologic	

Read pages 787-789 in your textbook; then answer questions 3 and 4.

3. The basic pathophysiology present in a woman with preeclampsia is _____ as

   a result of _____. As a result, blood flow to all organs may
   be diminished.

4. Match each of the signs or symptoms below with the preeclampsia-associated pathology it
   indicates. (*Note:* Some letters will be used more than once.)

   _____ Blurred vision/scotomata

   _____ Headache

   _____ Epigastric or right upper quadrant
            abdominal pain

   _____ 4+ reflexes/clonus

   _____ Elevated blood pressure

   _____ Proteinuria/oliguria

   a. Generalized vasoconstriction

   b. Glomerular damage

   c. Retinal arteriolar spasms

   d. Hepatic microemboli; liver damage

   e. Cortical brain spasms

Exercise 3

 CD-ROM Activity

 30 minutes

- Sign in to work at Pacific View Regional Hospital on the Obstetrics Floor for Period of Care 3. (*Note*: If you are already in the virtual hospital from a previous exercise, click on **Leave the Floor** and then **Restart the Program** to get to the sign-in window.)
- From the Patient List, select Kelly Brady.
- Click on **Go to Nurses' Station**.

 Read about HELLP syndrome on pages 788-789 in your textbook.

1. Why do you think Kelly Brady had blood drawn at 1230 for an AST measurement and a platelet count?

 - Click on **Chart** and then on **203**.
- Click on **Laboratory Reports**.
- Scroll to the report for Wednesday 1230 to locate the results of these tests.

 2. Complete the table below based on your review of the Laboratory Reports and Table 30-4 on page 792 in your textbook.

Test	Wed 1230 Result	Normal (Nonpregnant) Value	Value in HELLP
Platelet count			
AST			

 - Click on **Return to Nurses' Station**.
- Click on **Patient List**.
- In the far-right column click on **Get Report** for Kelly Brady.

3. Why has Kelly Brady been transferred to labor and delivery?

4. HELLP syndrome is not a separate illness, but a _____.

However, many women with HELLP syndrome may not have signs and symptoms of severe preeclampsia or may have only _____ in blood pressure. HELLP syndrome consists of _____, _____ enzymes, and _____.

HELLP syndrome is a _____ diagnosis.

5. What type of woman is most likely to develop HELLP syndrome? Which of these character-istics is true of Kelly Brady?

→ • Click on **Go to Nurses' Station.**
  • Click on **Chart** and then on **203**.
  • Click on **Physician's Notes**.
  • Scroll to the note for Wednesday 1530.

6. What is the physician's plan of care for Kelly Brady in light of the HELLP syndrome diagnosis?

Assume that you will be the nurse caring for Kelly Brady after her surgery while she is receiving magnesium sulfate. Read about this medication on pages 796-798 in your textbook and then answer question 7.

7. All of the assessments/interventions listed below are part of routine nursing care for a patient with severe preeclampsia. Place an X beside the activities that are performed specifi-cally to assess for magnesium toxicity.

_____ Measure/record urine output.

_____ Measure proteinuria using urine dipstick.

_____ Monitor liver enzyme levels and platelet count.

_____ Monitor for headache, visual disturbances, and epigastric pain.

_____ Assess for decreased level of consciousness.

_____ Assess DTRs.

_____ Weigh daily to assess for edema.

_____ Monitor vital signs, especially respiratory rate.

_____ Dim room lights and maintain a quiet environment.

13

Medical-Surgical Problems in Pregnancy

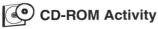 **Reading Assignment:** Medical-Surgical Problems in Pregnancy (Chapter 33)

Patients: Maggie Gardner, Room 204
Gabriela Valenzuela, Room 205

Goal: Demonstrate an understanding of the identification and management of selected medical-surgical problems in pregnancy.

Objectives:

- Identify appropriate interventions for managing selected medical-surgical problems in pregnancy.
- Plan and evaluate essential patient education during the acute phase of diagnosis.

Exercise 1

 CD-ROM Activity

 10 minutes

- Sign in to work at Pacific View Regional Hospital on the Obstetrics Floor for Period of Care 1. (*Note*: If you are already in the virtual hospital from a previous exercise, click on **Leave the Floor** and then **Restart the Program** to get to the sign-in window.)
- From the Patient List, select Gabriela Valenzuela.
- Click on **Go to Nurses' Station**.
- Click on **Chart** and then on **205**.
- Click on **History and Physical**.

Review material regarding cardiac problems during pregnancy on pages 849-852 in the textbook.

1. According to the textbook, 1%-4% of pregnancies are complicated with heart disease. In the History and Physical for Gabriela Valenzuela, what does the physician note as her cardiac problem?

2. Mitral valve disease is one of the most common causes of cardiac disease in pregnant women.
   a. True
   b. False

3. According to the History and Physical, what cardiac symptoms does Gabriela Valenzuela exhibit now that she is pregnant?

4. Based on your textbook reading, why do pregnant women with cardiac disorders have problems during their pregnancies?

5. What abnormal assessment finding is noted in the History and Physical that would be associated with Gabriela Valenzuela's cardiac disorder?

Exercise 2

 CD-ROM Activity

 20 minutes

 Autoimmune disorders encompass a wide variety of disorders that can be disruptive to the pregnancy process. Maggie Gardner in Room 204 has been admitted to rule out lupus. The following activities will explore the various aspects of this autoimmune disorder. First, review pages 869-870 in your textbook regarding systemic lupus erythematosus (SLE).

- Sign in to work at Pacific View Regional Hospital on the Obstetrics Floor for Period of Care 2. (*Note*: If you are already in the virtual hospital from a previous exercise, click on **Leave the Floor** and then **Restart the Program** to get to the sign-in window.)
- From the Patient List, select Maggie Gardner.
- Click on **Go to Nurses' Station**.
- Click on **Chart** and then on **204**.
- Click on **History and Physical**.

1. Based on Maggie Gardner's History and Physical, what information would correlate to a diagnosis of SLE?

2. According to the textbook, what is most often the presenting symptom of this disease during pregnancy?

- Click on **Return to Nurses' Station**.
- Click on Room **204** at the bottom of the screen.
- Click on **Patient Care** and then **Physical Assessment**.
- Click on various body areas (yellow buttons) and system subcategories (green buttons) to perform a head-to-toe assessment of Maggie Gardner. (*Hint:* Take notes during your assessment based on questions 3 and 4.)

3. Based on your head-to-toe assessment, list four abnormal findings that are related to Maggie Gardner's diagnosis.

- Click on **Chart** and then on **204**.
- Click on **Patient Education**.

4. Based on your physical assessment, the information from the Patient Education section of the chart, and the fact that this is a new diagnosis for the patient, list three areas of teaching that need to be completed with this patient.

Exercise 3

 CD-ROM Activity

 35 minutes

- Sign in to work at Pacific View Regional Hospital on the Obstetrics Floor for Period of Care 3. (*Note:* If you are already in the virtual hospital from a previous exercise, click on **Leave the Floor** and then **Restart the Program** to get to the sign-in window.)
- From the Patient List, select Maggie Gardner.
- Click on **Go to Nurses' Station**.
- Click on **Chart** and then **204**.

- Click on the **Consultations** tab.
- Review the Rheumatology Consult.

1. List four things that the rheumatologist notes in her impressions regarding specific findings that are associated with a diagnosis of SLE for Maggie Gardner.

→ • Click on **Diagnostic Reports**.

2. Maggie Gardner had an ultrasound done prior to the consult with the rheumatologist. What were the findings as they relate to SLE? What were the follow-up recommendations? (*Hint*: See Impressions section.)

3. What is the rheumatologist's plan regarding laboratory/diagnostics to gain a definitive diagnosis?

4. According to the Rheumatology Consult, what is the plan regarding medications (immediate need)?

- Click on **Return to Nurses' Station**.
- Click on the **Drug** icon in the lower left corner of the screen.
- Find the Drug Guide profile of prednisone. (*Hint:* You can type the drug name in the Search box or scroll through the alphabetic list of drugs at the top of the screen.)

5. What does Maggie Gardner need to be taught regarding this medication?

- Click on **Return to Nurses' Station**.
- Click on Room **204**.
- Click on **Patient Care** and then **Nurse-Client Interactions**.
- Select and view the video titled **1530: Disease Management**. (*Note:* Check the virtual clock to see whether enough time has elapsed. You can use the fast-forward feature to advance the time by 2-minute intervals if the video is not yet available. Then click on **Patient Care** and **Nurse-Client Interactions** to refresh the screen.)

6. During this video clip, the nurse provides Maggie Gardner with information regarding her disease. What two things does the nurse note that are important aspects of the patient's disease management during pregnancy?

7. What medication, ordered by the rheumatologist, will assist in the blood flow to the placenta? How?

8. What key component does the nurse identify for Maggie Gardner that will assist in maintaining a healthy pregnancy?

9. What excuse does Maggie Gardner give for not keeping previous doctor's appointments? (*Hint:* This information is found in the Nursing Admission in the chart.)

Exercise 4

 CD-ROM Activity

 15 minutes

- Sign in to work at Pacific View Regional Hospital on the Obstetrics Floor for Period of Care 4. (*Note*: If you are already in the virtual hospital from a previous exercise, click on **Leave the Floor** and then **Restart the Program** to get to the sign-in window.)
- From the Nurses' Station, click on **Chart** and then **204**. (*Remember:* You are not able to visit patients or administer medications during Period of Care 4. You are able to review patients' records only.)
- Click on **Laboratory Reports**.

1. The results are now available for the following laboratory tests that were ordered in Period of Care 2. What are the findings?

Laboratory Test	Result
C3	
C4	
CH50	
RPR	
ANA Titer	
Anticardiolipin	
Anti-sm; Anti-DNA; Anti–SSA	
Anti-SSB	
Anti-RVV; Antiphospholipid	

• Click on **Consultations** and review the Rheumatology Consult.

2. The lab findings you recorded in question 1 are definitive for the diagnosis of SLE. According to the textbook and the Rheumatology Consult, what is the plan to manage this disease once the baby is delivered?

 • Click on **Nurse's Notes.**

3. By Period of Care 4, Maggie Gardner has been provided with education regarding various aspects of her disease process, testing, and hospital procedures. Based on your review of the Nurse's Notes for Wednesday, what has she been specifically taught? Include the time each instruction took place.

4. Using correct NANDA nursing diagnosis terminology, write three possible nursing diagnoses for Maggie Gardner.

5. SLE requires long-term management because patients will experience remissions and exacerbations. What step did the rheumatologist take with Maggie Gardner to begin the long-term relationship that will be required to ensure a healthy outcome?

LESSON 14 ——————

Mental Health Disorders and Substance Abuse

👓 **Reading Assignment:** Mental Health Disorders and Substance Abuse (Chapter 35)

Patients: Kelly Brady, Room 203
Maggie Gardner, Room 204
Laura Wilson, Room 206

Goal: Demonstrate an understanding of the identification and management of selected mental health or substance abuse issues in pregnant women.

Objectives:

- Identify signs and symptoms of depression and anxiety in selected patients.
- Discuss the use of pharmacotherapy for treating depression and anxiety in pregnant and lactating patients.
- Assess and plan care for a substance abusing woman with a term pregnancy.

In this lesson you will assess and plan care for three pregnant women, all of whom have mental health or substance abuse problems.

Exercise 1

 CD-ROM Activity

 20 minutes

- Sign in to work at Pacific View Regional Hospital on the Obstetrics Floor for Period of Care 1. (*Note*: If you are already in the virtual hospital from a previous exercise, click on **Leave the Floor** and then **Restart the Program** to get to the sign-in window.)
- From the Patient List, select Kelly Brady.
- Click on **Go to Nurses' Station**.

 Read about Mood Disorders on pages 900-902 in your textbook.

137

1. List signs and symptoms associated with major depression.

2. In order to be diagnosed with _____, at least

   _____ of the signs/symptoms listed in question 1 must be present

   _____.

3. List risk factors for developing depression in pregnancy.

➤ • Click on **Go to Nurses' Station**.
  • Click on **Chart** and then on **203**.
  • Click on **Mental Health** and review the Psychiatric/Mental Health Assessment.

4. List Kelly Brady's signs/symptoms of major depression.

5. Does Kelly Brady meet the criteria for a diagnosis of major depression?

• Click on **Consultations**.

• Scroll to review the Psychiatric Consult, completed Tuesday at 1500.

6. Of the risk factors for developing depression during pregnancy listed in question 3, which are present in Kelly Brady's situation?

7. Using information from the Psychiatric Consult, list data that confirm the presence of the risk factors listed in question 6.

8. What is the management plan for Kelly Brady's depression recommended by the psychiatric consultant?

Read the section on Antidepressant Medications on pages 901-902 in your textbook.

9. What is the drug classification for paroxetine (Paxil)?

10. Kelly Brady plans to breastfeed her baby. How would you counsel her in regard to taking paroxetine (Paxil) while nursing? (*Hint*: Read the section on Medications and Breastfeeding on pages 730-731 in Chapter 27 of your textbook.)

 11. What suggestions would you give Kelly Brady to help prevent the development of postpartum depression? (*Hint*: See the Teaching for Self-Care box on page 917 in the textbook.)

Exercise 2

 CD-ROM Activity

 20 minutes

- Sign in to work at Pacific View Regional Hospital on the Obstetrics Floor for Period of Care 1. (*Note*: If you are already in the virtual hospital from a previous exercise, click on **Leave the Floor** and then **Restart the Program** to get to the sign-in window.)
- From the Patient List, select Maggie Gardner.
- Click on **Go to Nurses' Station**.
- Click on **Chart** and then on **204**.
- Click on **Nursing Admission**.

1. What are Maggie Gardner's admission diagnoses?

2. What seems to be the major cause of Maggie Gardner's anxiety?

3. Is Maggie Gardner's anxiety currently affecting her lifestyle? Support your answer using data from the Nursing Admission.

→ • Click on **History and Physical**.
   • Scroll to the OB History on page 2 of the History and Physical.

4. List Maggie Gardner's obstetric history, using the GTPAL format.

5. Based on Maggie Gardner's previous pregnancy history, why do you think she might be especially anxious at this particular time in her pregnancy?

→ • Click on **Physician's Orders**.
   • Scroll to the admission orders for Tuesday at 2115.

6. Identify the medication and dosage ordered specifically to treat Maggie Gardner's anxiety.

7. What important information is missing from the order in question 6? If you were the nurse caring for Maggie Gardner, how could you obtain this information?

• Click on **Return to Nurses' Station**.
• Click on **204** to go to the patient's room.
• Click on **Patient Care** and then **Nurse-Client Interactions**.
• Select and view the video titled **0745: Evaluation—Efficacy of Drugs**. (*Note:* Check the virtual clock to see whether enough time has elapsed. You can use the fast-forward feature to advance the time by 2-minute intervals if the video is not yet available. Then click on **Patient Care** and **Nurse-Client Interactions** to refresh the screen.)

8. How does Maggie Gardner describe her present emotional state?

9. Does Maggie Gardner believe the buspirone is helping to decrease her anxiety? Why or why not?

10. How does the nurse explain buspirone's effectiveness?

 • Click on the **Drug** icon in the lower left corner of the screen.
• Scroll down the drug list and click on **buspirone**.

11. Is Maggie Gardner's buspirone dosage appropriate?

12. Scroll down to read the Patient Teaching section in the Drug Guide. Based on this information, do you agree with the nurse's explanation about buspirone's effectiveness in the 0745 video? If not, how would you counsel Maggie Gardner about the effectiveness of this medication?

Exercise 3

 CD-ROM Activity

 20 minutes

• Sign in to work at Pacific View Regional Hospital on the Obstetrics Floor for Period of Care 2. (*Note:* If you are already in the virtual hospital from a previous exercise, click on **Leave the Floor** and then **Restart the Program** to get to the sign-in window.)

- From the Patient List, select Laura Wilson.
- Click on **Go to Nurses' Station**.
- Click on **Chart** and then on **206**.
- Click on **Nursing Admission**.

1. Complete the table by documenting Laura Wilson's use of alcohol and recreational drugs, based on your review of the Nursing Admission.

Substance	Reported Use
Tobacco	
Alcohol	
Marijuana	
Crack cocaine	

 Read about tobacco, alcohol, marijuana, and cocaine in the Substance Abuse During Pregnancy section on pages 904-907 in your textbook.

2. For each pregnancy-related risk listed in the table below, place an X under the substance(s) thought to be associated with that risk.

Pregnancy-Related Risk	Tobacco	Alcohol	Marijuana	Cocaine
Ectopic pregnancy				
Miscarriage				
Premature rupture of membranes				
Preterm birth				
Placenta previa				
Abruptio placentae				
Chorioamnionitis				
Fetal alcohol spectrum disorder (FASD)				
Hypertension				
Stillbirth				
Anemia				
Fetal abnormalities				

• Click on **Return to Nurses' Station**.
• Click on **206** at the bottom of the screen.
• Click on **Patient Care** and then **Nurse-Client Interactions**.
• Select and view the video titled **1115: Teaching—Effects of Drug Use**. (*Note:* Check the virtual clock to see whether enough time has elapsed. You can use the fast-forward feature to advance the time by 2-minute intervals if the video is not yet available. Then click on **Patient Care** and **Nurse-Client Interactions** to refresh the screen.)

3. Does Laura Wilson consider herself to be addicted? Support your answer with comments from the video.

4. How does Laura Wilson think her drug use will affect her baby?

5. According to the nurse in the video, how might Laura Wilson's drug use affect the baby?

Read the section on Plan of Care and Intervention on pages 910-912 in your textbook.

6. Assume that you are the nurse caring for Laura Wilson today. Which interventions to deal with Laura Wilson's drug use would be most appropriate at this time? Select all that apply.

_____ Talk with Laura Wilson in a manner that conveys caring and concern.

_____ Urge Laura Wilson to begin a drug treatment program today.

_____ Explain to Laura Wilson that she may lose custody of her baby if her drug use continues.

_____ Involve other members of the health care team in Laura Wilson's care.

7. Explain your choice(s) in question 6.

LESSON 15

Labor and Birth Complications

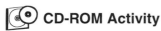 **Reading Assignment:** Labor and Birth Complications (Chapter 36)

Patients: Dorothy Grant, Room 201
Stacey Crider, Room 202
Kelly Brady, Room 203
Gabriela Valenzuela, Room 205

Goal: Demonstrate an understanding of the identification and management of selected labor and birth complications.

Objectives:

- Assess and identify signs and symptoms present in the patient with preterm labor.
- Describe appropriate nursing care for the patient in preterm labor.
- Develop a birth plan to meet the needs of the preterm infant.

In this lesson you will compare and contrast the care of four patients, all of whom are treated for preterm labor and/or will deliver preterm infants.

Exercise 1

 CD-ROM Activity

20 minutes

- Sign in to work at Pacific View Regional Hospital on the Obstetrics Floor for Period of Care 2. (*Note*: If you are already in the virtual hospital from a previous exercise, click on **Leave the Floor** and then **Restart the Program** to get to the sign-in window.)
- From the Patient List, select Dorothy Grant and Gabriela Valenzuela.
- Click on **Go to Nurses' Station**.
- Click on **Chart** and then on **201** for Dorothy Grant's chart.
- Click on **History and Physical**.

1. Using the information found in the History and Physical section, complete the table below for Dorothy Grant.

Patient	Weeks Gestation	Reason for Admission
Dorothy Grant		

- Click on **Return to Nurses' Station**.
- Now click again on **Chart**; this time, select **205** for Gabriela Valenzuela's chart.
- Click on **History and Physical**.

2. Using the information found in the History and Physical section, complete the table below for Gabriela Valenzuela.

Patient	Weeks Gestation	Reason for Admission
Gabriela Valenzuela		

- Click on **Return to Nurses' Station**.
- Click on **201** at the bottom of the screen to go to Dorothy Grant's room.
- Click on **Patient Care** and then **Physical Assessment**.
- Click on **Pelvic** and then on **Reproductive**.

3. Complete the table below with the results of Dorothy Grant's initial cervical examination.

Patient	Time	Dilation	Effacement	Station
Dorothy Grant				

- Click on **Return to Nurses' Station**.
- Click on **205** to go to Gabriela Valenzuela's room.
- Click on **Patient Care** and then **Physical Assessment**.
- Click on **Pelvic** and then on **Reproductive**.

4. Record the results of Gabriela Valenzuela's initial cervical examination in the table below.

Patient	Time	Dilation	Effacement	Station
Gabriela Valenzuela				

 Read the section on Early Recognition and Diagnosis of preterm labor on page 929 in your textbook.

5. What criteria are necessary in order to make a diagnosis of preterm labor?

6. As of Wednesday at 0800, would you consider both these patients to be in preterm labor? Give a rationale for your answer.

 Read the section on Tocolytics on pages 932-935 in your textbook to answer the following questions.

7. Would you recommend tocolytic therapy for Gabriela Valenzuela? Support your answer.

8. Match each of the medications below with the description of how it works as a tocolytic agent. (Letters may be used more than once.)

_____ Magnesium sulfate

_____ Nifedipine (Procardia)

_____ Ritodrine (Yutopar)

_____ Terbutaline (Brethine)

_____ Indomethacin (Indocin)

a. Inhibits calcium from entering smooth muscle cells, thus relaxing uterine contractions

b. Relaxes uterine smooth muscle as a result of stimulation of beta$_2$ receptors on uterine smooth muscle

c. Exact mechanism unclear, but promotes relaxation of smooth muscles

d. Suppresses preterm labor by blocking the production of prostaglandins

Exercise 2

CD-ROM Activity

30 minutes

- Sign in to work at Pacific View Regional Hospital on the Obstetrics Floor for Period of Care 1. (*Note*: If you are already in the virtual hospital from a previous exercise, click on **Leave the Floor** and then **Restart the Program** to get to the sign-in window.)
- From the Patient List, select Stacey Crider.
- Click on **Get Report**.

Stacey Crider was admitted yesterday in preterm labor and placed on magnesium sulfate. Her other admission diagnoses were bacterial vaginosis and gestational diabetes with poorly controlled blood glucose levels.

1. What is Stacey Crider's current status in regard to preterm labor?

 • Click on **Go to Nurses' Station**.
• Click on **Chart** and then on **202**.
• Click on **Physician's Orders**.
• Scroll to the orders for Wednesday at 0715.

2. Which of these orders relate specifically to Stacey Crider's diagnosis of preterm labor?

 • Scroll to the orders for Wednesday at 0730.

3. What medication changes are ordered?

 Read about terbutaline and nifedipine in Tocolytic Therapy for Preterm Labor Medication Guide (pages 933-935) in your textbook.

4. Why do you think Stacey Crider's physician changed his orders so quickly?

 • Click on **Return to Nurses' Station**.
• Click on **202** at the bottom of the screen.
• Inside the patient's room, click on **Take Vital Signs**.

5. What are Stacey Crider's vital signs at 0800?

Temperature

Pulse

Respirations

Blood pressure

6. Which of these parameters provides the most important information you would need prior to giving Stacey Crider's nifedipine dose? Why? (*Hint*: Read about nifedipine on pages 933-935 in your textbook.)

Like Dorothy Grant and Kelly Brady, Stacey Crider is also receiving betamethasone.

 Read about Promotion of Fetal Lung Maturity in your textbook on pages 935-936. Answer the following questions.

7. Why are all three of these patients receiving antenatal corticosteroid therapy?

8. What other benefits does this class of medication provide for preterm infants?

 • Click on **MAR**.
• Click on tab **202**.

9. What is Stacey Crider's ordered betamethasone dosage?

 10. How does this dosage compare with the recommended dosage listed in the Antenatal Corticosteroid Therapy with Betamethasone, Dexamethasone Medication Guide on page 936 of your textbook?

 • Click on **Return to Nurses' Station**.
• Click on **Medication Room**.
• Click on **Unit Dosage** and then drawer **202**.
• Click on **Betamethasone**.
• Click on **Put Medication on Tray** and then **Close Drawer**.
• Click on **View Medication Room**.

- Click on **Preparation**.
- Click on **Prepare** and follow the Preparation Wizard's prompts to complete preparation of Stacey Crider's betamethasone dose.
- Click on **Return to Medication Room**.
- Click on **202** to return to Stacey Crider's room.
- Click on **Check Armband** and then **Check Allergies**.
- Click on **Patient Care** and then **Medication Administration**.
- Find **Betamethasone** listed on the left side of your screen. To its right, click on the down arrow next to **Select** and choose **Administer**.
- Follow the Administration Wizard's prompts to administer Stacey Crider's betamethasone injection. Indicate **Yes** to document the injection in the MAR.
- Click on **Leave the Floor**.
- Click on **Look at Your Preceptor's Evaluation**.
- Click on **Medication Scorecard**. How did you do?

Exercise 3

 CD-ROM Activity

 30 minutes

- Sign in to work at Pacific View Regional Hospital on the Obstetrics Floor for Period of Care 4. (*Note*: If you are already in the virtual hospital from a previous exercise, click on **Leave the Floor** and then **Restart the Program** to get to the sign-in window.)
- Click on **Chart** and then **201**. (*Remember:* You are not able to visit patients or administer medications during Period of Care 4. You are able to review patients' records only.)
- Click on **Nurse's Notes**.
- Scroll to the note for Wednesday 1815.

1. Despite receiving terbutaline for tocolysis, Dorothy Grant's labor continues to progress. What are the findings from her cervical examination at this time?

 • Scroll to the note for Wednesday 1840. It states that Dorothy Grant is being prepped for delivery.

2. If you were the nurse caring for Dorothy Grant during delivery, what special preparations would you make to care for the baby immediately after birth?

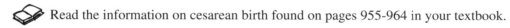

- Click on **Return to Nurses' Station**.
- Click again on **Chart**, but this time choose **205** for Gabriela Valenzuela's chart.
- Click on **Physician's Notes**.
- Scroll to the note for Wednesday 0800.

3. What is the anticipated outcome of Gabriela Valenzuela's labor, according to this note?

→ • Scroll to the notes for Wednesday 1415 and 1455.

4. What preparations have been made during the day for the birth of Gabriela Valenzuela's baby?

📖 Read the information on cesarean birth found on pages 955-964 in your textbook.

→ • Click on **Return to Nurses' Station**.
- Once again, click on **Chart**; select **203** for Kelly Brady's chart.
- Click on **Physician's Notes**.
- Scroll to the note for Wednesday 1530.

Kelly Brady was admitted yesterday with severe preeclampsia at 26 weeks gestation. Her preeclampsia is now worsening.

5. Why does her physician now recommend immediate delivery?

6. What general risks related to cesarean section does Kelly Brady's physician discuss with her?

7. Because of Kelly Brady's early gestational age (26 weeks), her physician anticipates a classical uterine incision. How will this type of incision affect Kelly Brady's birth options in future pregnancies?

• Click on **Physician's Orders**.
 • Scroll to the orders for Wednesday 1540.

8. List the orders to be carried out prior to Kelly Brady's surgery. State the purpose of each.

Order	Purpose

9. Can you think of other common preoperative procedures? List them below. (*Hint*: Refer to a basic Medical-Surgical textbook for ideas if you need help!)

LESSON **16** ————————————————————

Newborn Complications

✺ **Reading Assignment:** Acquired Problems of the Newborn (Chapter 38)
Nursing Care of the High-Risk Newborn (Chapter 40)

Patients: Stacey Crider, Room 202
Kelly Brady, Room 203
Gabriela Valenzuela, Room 205
Laura Wilson, Room 206

Goal: Demonstrate an understanding of the identification and management of selected common complications of newborns.

Objectives:

- Describe commonly occurring problems of infants of diabetic mothers.
- List nursing interventions related to hypoglycemia in infants of diabetic mothers.
- Identify risk factors for development of early-onset Group B strep infection and HIV infection.
- Describe common signs and symptoms of early-onset Group B strep infection.
- List nursing interventions for preventing transmission of the HIV virus to the neonate.
- Identify signs and symptoms of in-utero drug exposure in the neonate.
- Identify common problems found in extremely low-birth-weight infants.

In this lesson you will plan care for four newborns, all of whom are considered high-risk.

Exercise 1

 CD-ROM Activity

 20 minutes

- Sign in to work at Pacific View Regional Hospital on the Obstetrics Floor for Period of Care 4. (*Note*: If you are already in the virtual hospital from a previous exercise, click on **Leave the Floor** and then **Restart the Program** to get to the sign-in window.)
- Click on **Chart** and then on **202** for Stacey Crider's chart. (*Remember:* You are not able to visit patients or administer medications during Period of Care 4. You are able to review patients' records only.)
- Click on **History and Physical**.
- Scroll to History of Present Illness.

1. When was Stacey Crider's gestational diabetes diagnosed?

2. How was Stacey Crider's gestational diabetes managed?

 • Click on **Nursing Admission** and scroll to Diagnosis on page 1.

3. What was the status of Stacey Crider's gestational diabetes when she was admitted to the hospital at 27 weeks gestation?

 Assume that Stacey Crider has given birth and you are now the nurse caring for her baby. Read the section on Infants of Diabetic Mothers on pages 996-998 in your textbook.

4. Listed below are problems often seen in infants of diabetic mothers. Match each problem with the mechanism(s) responsible for that complication. (Answers may be used more than once.)

Problems	Responsible Mechanisms
_____ Congenital anomalies	a. Episodes of ketoacidosis
_____ Macrosomia	b. Fetal hyperinsulinemia
_____ Hypoglycemia	c. Maternal hyperglycemia
_____ Small-for-gestational-age (SGA) infant	d. Fluctuations in maternal blood glucose levels
_____ Respiratory distress syndrome	e. Maternal severe vascular disease

5. _____ is defined as a blood glucose level less than 40 mg/dL in a term infant.

Hypoglycemia most frequently manifests _____. Signs of

hypoglycemia include _____, _____, _____,

_____, and, in severe cases, _____.

 Consult the Plan of Care on page 1000 of your textbook.

6. List four nursing interventions to prevent or manage hypoglycemia in Stacey Crider's baby.

Exercise 2

 CD-ROM Activity

 30 minutes

Gabriela Valenzuela was admitted at 34 weeks gestation with vaginal bleeding and uterine contractions following an MVA. Her labor progressed throughout the day on Wednesday, and vaginal delivery is expected.

- Sign in to work at Pacific View Regional Hospital on the Obstetrics Floor for Period of Care 4. (*Note:* If you are already in the virtual hospital from a previous exercise, click on **Leave the Floor** and then **Restart the Program** to get to the sign-in window.)
- Click on **MAR** and then on tab **205** for Gabriela Valenzuela's records. (*Remember:* You are not able to visit patients or administer medications during Period of Care 4. You are able to review patients' records only.)

1. What medication has Gabriela Valenzuela been receiving today for Group B streptococcus prophylaxis?

- Click on **Return to Nurses' Station**.
- Click on **Chart** and then on **205**.
- Click on **Nurse's Notes**.
- Scroll to the note for Wednesday 1820.

2. What are the findings of Gabriela Valenzuela's cervical exam at this time?

Assume that Gabriela Valenzuela does give birth today. Read the Group B Streptococcus section on pages 1010-1011 in your textbook.

3. All of the following are risk factors for the development of early-onset GBS infection. Place an X beside the risk factor that you know would apply to Gabriela Valenzuela's baby.

_____ Low birth weight

_____ Preterm birth

_____ Rupture of membranes of more than 18 hours

_____ Maternal fever

_____ Previous infant with GBS infection

_____ Maternal GBS bacteriuria

_____ Multiple gestation

4. Early-onset GBS infection most commonly manifests _____.

Early-onset GBS infection usually results from _____ transmission from the

_____.

5. If you were the nurse caring for Gabriela Valenzuela's baby, what signs/symptoms might you see if the baby developed early-onset GBS?

Laura Wilson is a G1 P0 at 37 weeks gestation who is also HIV-positive. She was admitted last night with fever, vomiting, and diarrhea to rule out acute abdomen and pyelonephritis. During the day on Wednesday, Laura Wilson began having mild uterine contractions.

→ • From the Nurses' Station, click on **Chart** and then on **206**.
• Click on **Physician's Notes**.
• Scroll to the note for Wednesday at 0830.

6. Below, record Laura Wilson's HIV-related lab values.

CD4 count

HIV-1 RNA count

→ • Click on **Physician's Orders**.
• Scroll to the admission orders for Tuesday at 2130.

7. What is Laura Wilson's current antiretroviral drug regimen?

→ • Click on **Nurse's Notes**.
  • Scroll to the note for Wednesday 1830.

  8. What event occurred at 1815?

  9. Is Laura Wilson in labor at this time? Support your answer.

Laura Wilson is transferred to labor and delivery to give birth. Assume that she does give birth today. Read the section on Human Immunodeficiency Virus and Acquired Immunodeficiency Syndrome on pages 1006-1008 in your textbook.

  10. List factors that, if present, would increase the risk for transmission of HIV to Laura Wilson's baby during the birth process. Which risk factor does Laura Wilson have at this time?

  11. All infants born to seropositive mothers should be assumed to be _____. The

      accuracy of HIV testing in infants varies according to the _____ and is

      dependent on _____. The three methods currently used to

      detect HIV in neonates are _____, _____, and

      _____.

  12. What are the current testing recommendations for diagnosing HIV infection in newborns?

13. Assume that you are the nurse caring for Laura Wilson's baby in the newborn nursery. List nursing interventions to decrease the risk of viral transmission to the baby.

Exercise 3

 CD-ROM Activity

 15 minutes

In addition to being HIV-positive, Laura Wilson also has a past and current history of substance abuse.

- Sign in to work at Pacific View Regional Hospital on the Obstetrics Floor for Period of Care 4. (*Note*: If you are already in the virtual hospital from a previous exercise, click on **Leave the Floor** and then **Restart the Program** to get to the sign-in window.)
- Click on **Chart** and then on **206** for Laura Wilson's chart. (*Remember:* You are not able to visit patients or administer medications during Period of Care 4. You are able to review patients' records only.)
- Click on **Nursing Admission**.

1. Complete the chart below with information on Laura Wilson's current use of alcohol and recreational drugs (found on page 4 of the Nursing Admission).

Substance	Reported Use
Alcohol	
Marijuana	
Crack cocaine	

 Read about alcohol, marijuana, and cocaine in the Substance Abuse section on pages 1012-1017 in your textbook.

2. Listed below are problems often seen in infants exposed prenatally to alcohol, marijuana, or cocaine. Indicate the substance(s) thought to be associated with each problem by marking an X in the proper column(s). (*Note:* More than one drug may be associated with each problem.)

Problem	Alcohol	Marijuana	Cocaine
Craniofacial abnormalities			
Intrauterine growth restriction (IUGR)			
Hyperactivity			
Congenital anomalies			
Developmental delay			
Hypersensitivity to noise and external stimuli			
Difficult to console			

3. Fetal alcohol syndrome (FAS) is based on minimal criteria of signs in each of three

   categories: _____,

   _____, and _____. A baby who

   has been affected by prenatal exposure to alcohol but does not meet the criteria for FAS

   may be said to have an _____ or _____.

Read the Nursing Care section on pages 1017-1020 in your textbook.

4. List several appropriate interventions for the nurse assigned to work with Laura Wilson as she learns to accept and care for her drug-exposed baby.

Exercise 4

 CD-ROM Activity

 20 minutes

Kelly Brady was admitted with severe preeclampsia at 26 weeks gestation. Because of worsening maternal condition, she gives birth on Wednesday by cesarean section.

- Sign in to work at Pacific View Regional Hospital on the Obstetrics Floor for Period of Care 4. (*Note*: If you are already in the virtual hospital from a previous exercise, click on **Leave the Floor** and then **Restart the Program** to get to the sign-in window.)
- Click on **Chart** and then on **203** for Kelly Brady's chart. (*Remember:* You are not able to visit patients or administer medications during Period of Care 4. You are able to review patients' records only.)
- Click on **Diagnostic Reports**.

  1. According to the ultrasound done on Tuesday, what is Kelly Brady's baby's estimated fetal weight?

 - Click on **Consultations**.
- Review the Neonatology Consult for Wednesday at 0800.

  2. List common problems for babies born at 26 weeks gestation at Pacific View Regional Hospital, according to the neonatologist who met with Kelly Brady and her husband.

Read the section on Assessment and Nursing Diagnoses on pages 683-684 in Chapter 26 in your textbook.

3. If Kelly Brady's baby's actual weight is close to her estimated weight, in which weight category will she be placed? Why?

 Now read the section on Assessment and Nursing Diagnoses on pages 1054-1056 in your textbook.

4. Many body systems or functions are likely to be impaired in VLBW infants. Place an X beside the systems or functions that were also addressed by the neonatologist during his consultation with Kelly Brady. (*Hint:* See your answer to question 2.)

_____ Respiratory function

_____ Cardiovascular function

_____ Maintenance of body temperature

_____ CNS function

_____ Maintenance of adequate nutrition

_____ Maintenance of renal function

_____ Maintenance of hematologic status

_____ Resistance to infection

 Read the section on Parental Adaptation to Preterm Infant on pages 1057-1058 in your textbook.

5. List several psychologic tasks which Kelly Brady and/or her husband must accomplish as parents.

6. Write a nursing diagnosis appropriate for the Bradys, as parents of a premature baby who will have an extended NICU stay. (*Hint*: Consult the Plan of Care on pages 1072-1073 in the textbook.)

 7. List several nursing interventions to assist the Bradys in accomplishing the parenting tasks you listed in question 5. (*Hint*: Consult the Plan of Care on pages 1072-1073 in the text-book.)

LESSON 17

Grieving the Loss of a Newborn

Reading Assignment: Grieving the Loss of a Newborn (Chapter 41)

Patient: Maggie Gardner, Room 204

Goal: Demonstrate an understanding of the grieving process and how it relates to coping with a current pregnancy.

Objectives:

- Identify the various types of loss as they relate to a pregnancy.
- Describe the stages and phases of the grieving process.
- Identify various methods of coping exhibited by patients who have experienced the loss of a newborn.

Exercise 1

Writing Activity

 10 minutes

 Review pages 1091-1092 in the textbook.

1. Parents may grieve not only the death of a newborn but also the birth of a baby with a

   _____ or _____.

2. List other times that couples may grieve a loss related to pregnancy.

3. Women experience what type of effects if a pregnancy ends early due to miscarriage?

4. Miscarriages occur in _____ of all pregnancies.

5. Grief involves _____ and related _____ and _____ responses to a major loss.

6. All women and men who undergo a loss receive the support that they need.
   a. True
   b. False

Exercise 2

CD-ROM Activity

10 minutes

- Sign in to work at Pacific View Regional Hospital on the Obstetrics Floor for Period of Care 4. (*Note*: If you are already in the virtual hospital from a previous exercise, click on **Leave the Floor** and then **Restart the Program** to get to the sign-in window.)
- Click on **Chart** and then on **204** for Maggie Gardner's chart. (*Remember*: You are not able to visit patients or administer medications during Period of Care 4. You are able to review patients' records only.)
- Review the **History and Physical**.

1. How many losses related to pregnancy has Maggie Gardner experienced?

- Click on the **Nursing Admission**.

2. What is the first evidence you find that Maggie Gardner's previous losses are affecting her current pregnancy and care? (*Hint*: Review the first five sections.)

- Click on the **Consultations** tab.

3. To what does Maggie Gardner attribute her inability to have a child?

4. List three therapeutic measures the chaplain can use to assist her through these feelings as part of her grieving process?

5. What did the chaplain accomplish during his time with Maggie Gardner?

Exercise 3

CD-ROM Activity

15 minutes

Review pages 1091-1096 in your textbook.

1. What is grief?

2. What are the four tasks of grief?

3. What are the three phases of grief?

4. Mothers are the focus during the loss of an infant; however, the _____ shares

the _____ level of grief.

5. What response typically emerges during intense grief? Why?

6. List three other emotions that are experienced during the time period of intense grief.

7. During the phase of reorganization, what is the most common question? Explain.

 • Sign in to work at Pacific View Regional Hospital on the Obstetrics Floor for Period of Care 4. (*Note:* If you are already in the virtual hospital from a previous exercise, click on **Leave the Floor** and then **Restart the Program** to get to the sign-in window.)

• Click on **Chart** and then on **204**. (*Remember:* You are not able to visit patients or administer medications during Period of Care 4. You are able to review patients' records only.)

• Review the **History and Physical**.

8. You have now reviewed Maggie Gardner's History and Physical and compared her information with your textbook's discussion of what happens during the reorganization phase. What correlation do you see?

 • Click on **Consultations**.

• Scroll down to review the Pastoral Care Spiritual Assessment.

9. Culture and religion play very large roles in how individuals handle a loss. How has Maggie Gardner handled her losses? (*Hint*: See the Spirituality/Faith Factors section of this consult.)

LESSON **18** ─────────────────────

Medication Administration

Patients: Dorothy Grant, Room 201
Stacey Crider, Room 202
Maggie Gardner, Room 204
Laura Wilson, Room 206

Goal: Correctly administer selected medications to obstetric patients.

Objective:

- Correctly administer selected medications to obstetric patients, observing the Five Rights.

In this lesson you will give medications to selected obstetrics patients, observing the Five Rights.

Exercise 1

 CD-ROM Activity

 30 minutes

Dorothy Grant was admitted at 30 weeks gestation for observation following blunt abdominal trauma (she was kicked in the abdomen). She is bleeding vaginally and may have sustained a placental abruption. Your assignment for this exercise is to give Rh immune globulin to Dorothy Grant.

- Sign in to work at Pacific View Regional Hospital on the Obstetrics Floor for Period of Care 2. (*Note*: If you are already in the virtual hospital from a previous exercise, click on **Leave the Floor** and then **Restart the Program** to get to the sign-in window.)
- From the Patient List, select Dorothy Grant.

Read about Rh immune globulin on pages 603-604 in your textbook.

1. Rh immune globulin is a solution of _____ that contains _____.

    Rh immune globulin is given to _____

    who has had a _____.

    Rh immune globulin prevents sensitization by _____

    _____.

2. All of the following are reasons that Rh immune globulin might be administered. Place an X beside the reason it has been ordered for Dorothy Grant.

    _____   Within 72 hours of giving birth to an Rh-positive infant

    _____   Prophylactically at 28 weeks gestation

    _____   Following an incident or exposure risk that occurs after 28 weeks gestation

    _____   During first trimester pregnancy following miscarriage or elective abortion or ectopic pregnancy

3. List the information about Dorothy Grant that must be determined before giving her Rh immune globulin.

→ • Click on **Go to Nurses' Station**.
   • Click on **Chart** and then on **201**.
   • Click on **Physician's Orders**.
   • Scroll to the orders for Wednesday 0730.

4. Write the physician's order for Rh immune globulin.

5. According to your textbook, is this the correct dosage and route?

→ • Click on **Laboratory Reports**.
   • Locate the results for 0245 Wednesday.
   • Scroll down to find the type and screen results.

6. Dorothy Grant's blood type is _____.

7. What additional information do you need? Why? Is that information available?

 • Click on **Return to Nurses' Station**.
 • Click on **Medication Room**.
 • Click on **Refrigerator**; then click on the refrigerator door to open it.
 • Click on **Put Medication on Tray** and then on **Close Door**.
 • Click on **View Medication Room**.
 • Click on **Preparation**.
 • Click on **Prepare** and follow the prompts to complete preparation of this medication.
 • Click on **Return to Medication Room**.
 • Click on **201** to go to Dorothy Grant's room.
 • Click on **Check Armband**.
 • Click on **Patient Care** and then **Medication Administration**.

You are almost ready to give Dorothy Grant's injection. However, before you do . . .

8. Rh immune globulin is often considered a blood product.
   a. True
   b. False

9. Suppose Dorothy Grant tells you that because of her religious beliefs, she absolutely refuses to accept blood or blood products. How would you handle the situation?

Now you're ready to administer the medication!

 • Click on the down arrow next to **Select**; choose **Administer**.
 • Follow the prompts to administer Dorothy Grant's injection. Indicate **Yes** to document the injection in the MAR.
 • Click on **Leave the Floor**.
 • Click on **Look at Your Preceptor's Evaluation**.
 • Click on **Medication Scorecard**. How did you do?

Exercise 2

 CD-ROM Activity

 20 minutes

- Sign in to work at Pacific View Regional Hospital on the Obstetrics Floor for Period of Care 1. (*Note*: If you are already in the virtual hospital from a previous exercise, click on **Leave the Floor** and then **Restart the Program** to get to the sign-in window.)
- From the Patient List, select Maggie Gardner.
- Click on **Go to Nurses' Station**.
- Click on the **Chart** and then on **204**.
- Click on the **Nursing Admission**.

1. Maggie Gardner verbalizes anxiety repeatedly throughout the Nursing Admission. What is her primary concern? Why? Provide documentation.

2. Maggie Gardner states that prior to this pregnancy she had a highly adaptive coping mechanism. How does she consider her ability to cope at this point? Why? (*Hint*: See the Coping and Stress Tolerance section in the Nursing Admission.)

 • Click on the **Physician's Orders**.

3. What medication has the physician ordered to help Maggie Gardner with her anxiety?

 • Click on **Return to Room 204**.
- Click on **Nurses' Station**.
- Click on the **Drug** icon in the lower-left corner of your screen.
- Use the Search box or the scroll bar to find the medication you identified in question 3.
- Review all of the information provided regarding this drug.

4. What is the drug's mechanism of action?

- Click on **Return to Nurses' Station**.
- Click on **204** to go to Maggie Gardner's room.
- Click on **Patient Care** and then **Nurse-Client Interactions**.
- Select and view the video titled **0745: Evaluation—Efficacy of Drugs**. (*Note:* Check the virtual clock to see whether enough time has elapsed. You can use the fast-forward feature to advance the time by 2-minute intervals if the video is not yet available. Then click on **Patient Care** and **Nurse-Client Interactions** to refresh the screen.)

5. According to the nurse, how long will it take for Maggie Gardner to see therapeutic effects? How does this correlate with what you learned in the Teaching Section of the Drug Guide?

Exercise 3

 CD-ROM Activity

 15 minutes

In this exercise, you will administer betamethasone to Stacey Crider, who was admitted to the hospital at 27 weeks gestation in preterm labor.

- Sign in to work at Pacific View Regional Hospital on the Obstetrics Floor for Period of Care 1. (*Note*: If you are already in the virtual hospital from a previous exercise, click on **Leave the Floor** and then **Restart the Program** to get to the sign-in window.)
- From the Patient List, select Stacey Crider.

1. Before preparing Stacey Crider's betamethasone, what do you need to do first?

- Click on **Go to Nurses' Station**.
- Click on **Chart** and then on **202**.
- Click on **Physician's Orders**.
- Scroll until you find the order for betamethasone.

2. After verifying the physician's order, what's your next step?

- Click on **Return to Nurses' Station**.
- Click on **Medication Room**.
- Click on **Unit Dosage** and then drawer **202**.
- Click on **Betamethasone**.
- Click on **Put Medication on Tray** and then **Close Drawer**.
- Click on **View Medication Room**.
- Click on **Preparation**.
- Click on **Prepare** and follow the prompts to complete preparation of Stacey Crider's betamethasone dose.
- Click on **Return to Medication Room**.

3. Now that the medication is prepared, what's your next step?

- Click on **202** to go to the patient's room.
- Click on **Check Armband** and then **Check Allergies**.
- Click on **Patient Care** and then **Medication Administration**.
- Click on the down arrow next to **Select** and choose **Administer**.
- Follow the prompts to administer Stacey Crider's betamethasone injection.

4. What's the final step in the process?

- If you haven't already, indicate **Yes** to document the injection in the MAR.
- Click on **Leave the Floor**.
- Click on **Look at Your Preceptor's Evaluation**.
- Click on **Medication Scorecard**. How did you do?

Exercise 4

 CD-ROM Activity

 30 minutes

- Sign in to work at Pacific View Regional Hospital on the Obstetrics Floor for Period of Care 1. (*Note*: If you are already in the virtual hospital from a previous exercise, click on **Leave the Floor** and then **Restart the Program** to get to the sign-in window.)
- From the Patient List, select Laura Wilson.
- Click on **Go to Nurses' Station**.
- Click on **MAR**.
- Click on the tab for Room **206**.

1. Laura Wilson's medications for Wednesday include several different types of drugs. In the list below, place an X next to the one that is used to treat her HIV-positive status.

   _____   Zidovudine 200 mg po every 8 hours

   _____   Prenatal multivitamin 1 tablet po daily

   _____   Lactated Ringer's 1000 mL IV continuous

- Click on **Return to Nurses' Station**.
- Click on the **Drug** icon in the lower-left corner of the screen.
- Using the Search box or the scroll bar, find the drug you identified in question 1.

2. What is the drug's mechanism of action?

3. What is the drug's therapeutic effect?

4. Does this medication cross the placenta? Is it distributed in breast milk?

5. What symptoms/side effects of this medication need to be reported to the physician?

6. How should this medication be taken?

7. As a final assignment you are to give Laura Wilson the medication that is due at 0800. During these lessons, we have provided you with the detailed instructions on how to give medications. Now it is time for you to fly solo. If you are administering the medication from the last question, start by clicking on **Return to Nurses' Station**. Don't forget the Five Rights of medication administration . . . and have fun!! Document below how you did.

If you'd like to get more practice, there are other medications that can be given at the beginning of the first three periods of care. Below is a list of the patients, the medications, the routes of administration, and the administration times you can use. As you practice, be sure to select the correct patient when you sign in. That way, you can get a Medication Scorecard for evaluation after you prepare and administer a medication. (*Remember:* If you need help at any time, refer to pages 22, 26-30, and 36-40 in the **Getting Started** section of this workbook.)

PERIOD OF CARE 1

Room 201, Dorothy Grant

0730/0800

Betamethasone 12 mg IM

Prenatal multivitamin PO

Room 202, Stacey Crider

0800—Prenatal multivitamin PO

Metronidazole 500 mg PO

Betamethasone 12 mg IM

Insulin lispro Sub-Q

Nifedipine 20 mg PO

Room 203, Kelly Brady

0730/0800—Prenatal multivitamin PO

Ferrous sulfate PO

Labetalol hydrochloride 400 mg PO

Nifedipine 10 mg PO

Room 204, Maggie Gardner

0800—Prenatal multivitamin PO

Buspirone hydrochloride 5 mg PO

Room 205, Gabriela Valenzuela

0800—Ampicillin 2 g IV

Betamethasone 12 mg IM

Prenatal multivitamin PO

Room 206, Laura Wilson

0800—Zidovudine 200 g PO

Prenatal multivitamin PO

PERIOD OF CARE 2

Room 201, Dorothy Grant

1200—Rho(D) immune globulin IM

Room 202, Stacey Crider

1200—Insulin lispro Sub-Q

Room 203, Kelly Brady

1130—Betamethasone 12 mg IM

Room 204, Maggie Gardner

1115—Prednisone 40 mg PO

Aspirin 81 mg PO

PERIOD OF CARE 3

Room 204, Maggie Gardner

1500—Buspirone 5 mg PO

Notes:

Notes:

Notes: